THE DOOR OPENS

A door opens ahead of me—a new experience. I find myself a confusion of feelings, a mingling of anticipation and fear.

How shall I prepare myself for this forward step?

The temptation is to weigh myself down with everything that I was yesterday, to protect myself with the armor of past thoughts and feelings. But what lies ahead is more than yesterday or even today could ever be, and if I am loaded down with what I was, how will I be able to be what I am?

Alex Noble

Uniquely You

BETTY NETHERY
& BEVERLY BUSH SMITH

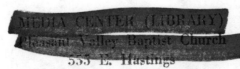
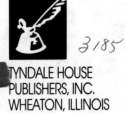
TYNDALE HOUSE
PUBLISHERS, INC.
WHEATON, ILLINOIS

Quotes from the booklet, "You Are Really Somebody," by J. Allan Petersen, are used by permission of Family Concern, Box 419, Wheaton, Ill. 60189.

All Scripture references are taken from *The New International Version* unless otherwise indicated.

First printing, February 1984
Library of Congress Catalog Card Number 83-51176
ISBN 0–8423–7792–1

CONTENTS

FOREWORD

True inward and outward beauty are almost impossible to separate, since one almost always echoes the other. As Betty Nethery, founder of Uniquely You®, works with women, she finds that helping them look better can literally change their lives, because it changes their inward feelings about themselves. But most of us recognize that what is inside us also shines through outwardly. Often, for instance, there is a dramatic change in appearance, a softening of features, a glow which comes when someone begins to know the true source of inner peace and security.

Betty first approached me with the idea of writing a book to help women achieve harmony in their appearance, no matter what their age, shape, or size—to demonstrate that any woman can look wonderful. This is what she teaches in her popular and effective Uniquely You seminars.

But because I see Betty as personally possessing both inner and outer beauty, I urged that we not simply add another narcissistic worship-of-self book to the market, but that we reach deeper. After all, true beauty is not skin deep or bone deep; it goes clear to the soul.

Betty agreed enthusiastically, but we soon found we had not undertaken a simple task. This book underwent many, many revisions, as we worked to intertwine these two facets of beauty and to express them in a manner which would touch as many lives as possible.

Through it all, my own personal role model has been the biblical Sarah, who demonstrates this balance. She was so physically beautiful that her husband twice presented her as his sister because he was so afraid other men would desire her and want to kill him. Yet in the New Testament, Sarah is celebrated as a woman of great inner beauty, a woman of faith (Hebrews 11:11) and a woman who "hoped in God" and "adorned herself with a gentle and quiet spirit" (1 Peter 3:1–6).

This book, then, comes to you in the hope that we may grow to be like Sarah. It is my prayer that we may be grounded in the inner beauty which springs from a growing knowledge of God, from sharing and drawing from his very nature; and, at the same time, that we may achieve our own personal outward beauty as his totally unique creation.

INTRODUCTION

This book is actually my own personal life's lesson. I frequently tell
the women and men who attend our Uniquely You seminars across
the country that we all tend to teach what we ourselves need to
learn. I wanted to *learn* to be attractive. In this book I am sharing
the ideas and helps I've been developing since 1977, when I founded
Uniquely You, a consulting firm to help people develop their own
image.

You see, as a child, I was a model; but as a pre-adolescent, I
couldn't believe what had happened to that "model child." I was
too tall, too thin, too bony; I was miserable. No wonder boys didn't
pay any attention to me!

At thirteen, I drew closer to God and made a decision to follow
him, and to trust that he would direct me to fulfill all that I was
capable of. And although I still felt rejected by my peers, I found a
new sense of identity, an assurance in being so totally acceptable
that there was a purpose for my life.

But I still felt I *looked* like a frump.

In college, I had a friend who owned only three outfits, but used
them so cleverly, she seemed to have a closet full of clothes. She
began teaching me how to look my very best. However, it took
years and years of struggling and trial and error before I began to
understand how to work with my body, features, and coloring. But,
at last—the feeling of having achieved a total look which was right
for me was wonderful!

In the following years, I experienced a number of extremes: from
devoting all my time to sharing my faith, to feeling Christianity was
too oppressively full of "have-to's"; from feeling totally unlovely, to
concentrating all my efforts on being just as attractive as I could.

So I've had to learn—and I am still learning—how to balance
outer attractiveness with that inner beauty referred to in 1 Peter
3:4.

The word *beauty*, I must confess, makes me a bit nervous. But I know of no other which conveys the excellence I feel we all, deep down, long to achieve. And I truly believe that every woman can choose to be beautiful and learn to be beautiful, just as the biblical Sarah was, both inside and out.

I feel a need to be careful, however, to keep this quest in proportion, so we won't imitate Rachel or Bathsheba, whose beauty did not go clear to the soul. And we must also be aware of the pitfall of pride, which could cause us to see beauty as our own, rather than as a gift and an expression of God's own nature.

The world tends to judge, "Now, she is beautiful; and she is not."

This really is not so. Yet for us to simply "want to be beautiful" is a bit like wanting to be "happy." It doesn't just happen. We must make it happen by learning certain basics, taking specific steps. It's a continuing process. (Yes, you can become more beautiful as you grow older!)

Remember how God taught his chosen people exactly how his tabernacle should be adorned? He specified every tiny detail of size, shape, and color. Well, have you considered that our bodies are the temples of God when he is a living part of us? We can learn to adorn our temples in a way which says to the world, "Here is a woman who loves and honors God."

But how do we define beauty? It's a bit like defining love, for true beauty is so complex, so subject to personal preferences and cultures. Still, certain facets of beauty seem universal.

Beauty is perspective. It is a way of representing objects or viewing them, so that some parts appear closer and more important and others appear more distant and less important. Perspective gives a sense of proportion, a sense of values. We could photograph Notre Dame Cathedral from one *perspective* if we stood in the street in front of it. But we'd have quite a different perspective if we went inside and focused upon the light streaming through a stained glass window.

In this book, we'll discuss God's perspective of us—how he sees us—and how we can learn to see ourselves realistically, and appreciate our own bodies, with their unique shapes and proportions.

Beauty is style—not fashion, with its ephemeral dictates, but rather, a particular manner or form of presentation. Beauty should reflect a manner which is characteristic of a person—it should be the true and honest expression of a person's uniqueness. In music, the dreamy flow of Debussy is distinct in *style*, as contrasted with the storm and thunder of Wagner.

In chapter 3, we'll focus on recognizing your own personal inner style or gifts, as well as your personal style preferences in clothing.

Beauty is harmony, with different elements working together in a pleasant, connected, homogenous whole. It is the discarding of discordant parts which jar or distract. You hear harmony when everyone in a vocal ensemble sings the proper notes. But if just one member is a tad off-key, it sets your teeth on edge, because that person has spoiled the *harmony* of the presentation.

In chapter 4, we deal with the harmony of God's plan for our lives, and how to recognize the harmony of his color plan for us.

Beauty is contrast or the placing of two dissimilar elements so that the one heightens the differences and the effect of the other. In a Beethoven symphony, the slow movement contrasts with and heightens the beauty of the scherzo. In a Rembrandt painting, the highlights stand in radiant contrast to the depth of the shadows.

Chapter 5 addresses the contrasts of the way we were created as men and women, and shows you how to look radiantly and wonderfully feminine.

Beauty is attention to details, so that the smaller elements work together to enhance the whole. It means coordinating carefully, always evaluating. In Michelangelo's famous "David," the stance of the figure, the position of the head, each curve, each line, every *detail* works together to create a statue of magnificent strength and beauty.

Chapter 6, then, looks at God's caring for every detail of your life, and how you can carefully bring together all the details of your appearance, from accessories, to your hair and makeup.

Beauty is eliminating. It is the discarding of that which is not significant in order to concentrate and focus upon more important elements. When Matisse designed his murals for the chapel in Vence, France, he drew enormously detailed preliminary sketches. Then he eliminated and concentrated. In the end, just a few lines tell us everything.

So in chapter 7, we take inventory, both internally and externally, seeking to get rid of the old "data" which cripples our lives, as well as the unneeded and unflattering clothes which tend to clutter our closets.

Beauty is design. There must be a plan or structure for any building, any piece of music or art. It would be impossible for the Washington Cathedral to look so pleasing, or, indeed, to stand at all, without a design.

In chapter 8, then, we focus on a foundation for building or re-building our lives, and on a design for rebuilding our wardrobes.

Perhaps most of all, *beauty is communication; it is a statement,* a reaching out which is designed to be meaningfully perceived by another person. Thus, while a Toulouse-Lautrec poster may speak of the decadence of Paris night life, a Bach cantata is a clear communication of the purity and glory of God.

So, at the very beginning of this book, we consider what you are saying—how messages flow to others from your innermost being, and how the language of your appearance speaks to others.

As we think of all these facets of beauty, we tend to view them in terms of the eye (or ear) of the beholder. But as I think about them, I realize they are also qualities which Christ embodies!

For he truly is the ultimate in beauty. And I am overwhelmed when I consider that it is our magnificent destiny to become like him.

Betty Nethery

BEAUTY IS COMMUNICATION

1

WHAT ARE YOU SAYING?

"When I first met Linda, I thought she was one of the most beautiful women I'd ever seen," a young man told me recently. "But as I began talking with her, I soon realized how negative she was about everything, how centered on herself. After awhile she wasn't even pretty anymore."

Perhaps you've had a similar experience of initially admiring someone's astonishing good looks, but then finding that person so lacking in inner resources that he or she no longer seemed attractive to you.

Potiphar's wife and Rachel in the Bible are excellent examples of skin-deep beauty which does not endure; the unattractiveness *will* come through.

The opposite is also true. A client came to me recently for consultation, and when she walked in the door, I thought she was surely the most unattractive woman I'd ever seen. Large-boned and ungainly, she would never weigh less than 150 pounds. She had a huge nose, tiny mouth, sunken jaw, and was already undergoing electrolysis treatment for facial hair. She wanted a "complete makeover," and was considering plastic surgery.

But as we sat and talked and she relaxed and told me about herself, her boyfriend, her faith, all the warmth and love that was within her began to shine through. I no longer saw her as unattractive.

I saw a similar phenomenon at a church mother-daughter celebration. I assumed that since the woman in blue wore a corsage, she must be our speaker, but I couldn't help but think, as she sipped coffee beforehand, how pale and plain she appeared.

Later, when she stepped to the platform, looked out at us, and smiled, I gasped at the change. Her face became radiant.

What could account for this transformation? I think it was her inner beauty which suddenly shone through and continued to glow as she revealed her love of the Lord in her face, her body language, and the words of her powerful message.

Have you thought about what qualities of your innermost being shine through to others? Take a good look in your mirror. What do you see? What does your face say to others about your priorities, your attitudes, your outlook?

Does your face disclose

joy or melancholy?
sensitivity or hardness?
kindness or selfishness?
humility or arrogance?
gentleness or harshness?
patience or impatience?
love or hate?

Most of us would love to mirror the attributes in the left-hand column, but I've found that our natural tendency seems to be to choose the negative.

Recently, to my surprise, a woman asked me to be her mentor. She said she wanted to learn how to be more sensitive in dealing with people, how to keep cool in the midst of storms.

Well, I believe that if, indeed, I demonstrate either of those traits, it is because of the presence of Jesus within me. For wouldn't you agree that, in all of history, he is the greatest example of all those qualities? He is the source, the well-spring in us.

This is what I believe I saw in that speaker. It is the phenomenon known as Christ within. Paul expressed this mystery when he wrote, "It is no longer I who live, but Christ who lives in me ... I live by faith in the Son of God, who loved me and gave himself for me" (Galatians 2:20).

When he is part of us, then, we can put on those qualities as part of a new "inner wardrobe." Colossians 3:12–14 speaks of "clothing ourselves with compassion, kindness, humility, gentleness and patience," of being forgiving and of "putting on" love, which binds the other attributes together in perfect unity.

How do some of these traits look in day-to-day living? We see compassion when a friend comes to us in our grief, puts an arm around us, and hurts with us—weeps with us. We see kindness when a child interrupts a busy mother, and that mother stops to give the child her complete attention. We see humility when Karen allows Nancy to be praised for her work, though Karen's as good at it, or better. We see gentleness when a husband softly strokes the face of his desperately ill wife. And we find patience when a family listens to an aged parent's favorite joke for the ninety-ninth time—and laughs appreciatively.

The way we can show what's within, is to *do* and to view situations (which we might be inclined to perceive negatively) as opportunities to show forth Christ's love.

And the key to this "show and flow" is to focus, not on ourselves, but on him.

How can we do this?

One way might be to look for his presence all around us, in nature. As I walk along the stream below our house, I love to focus on his beauty on every side, to praise and thank him. It helps me keep my perspective in the midst of a very full schedule.

I also rely on the support of my friends. It is they who uphold me and encourage me with gentle reminders, such as "Don't you think God is big enough to handle that?" or, "Won't it be exciting to see how God will work this situation out?"

Won't you stop a moment to consider where your focus is today and how it is reflected? What inner resources shine through to others? Ask your friends and family for feedback on what they see—and are tired of seeing. What messages flow out to them about your outlook, your basis for living, the well-being of your mind and heart and spirit?

Earlier in this chapter we talked about how we can look past or through an outer unattractiveness to an inner beauty. However, I think some of us who are followers of Christ can become so focused on the inner that we neglect the outer. Is this good management of the bodies God created to be his temples, and entrusted to us?

Now, certainly, we don't want to place more emphasis upon the outer than on the inner, imperishable qualities of "a gentle and quiet spirit" (1 Peter 3:3).

But I urge you to consider that presenting ourselves as attractively as possible is not frivolous or superficial. Rather, it makes us accessible to others, opens opportunities for us to interface with them.

Because beauty, you remember, is a communication, a statement, both from within and without. Our mind continuously receives messages from what we see. Let's look, then, at

THE LANGUAGE OF YOUR APPEARANCE

Does your appearance make a positive statement to the world?
Do you ever feel that people fail to take you seriously?
Do your clothing styles reflect the "real you?"
Are you getting the treatment or service you feel you deserve?
"Why should it matter what I wear? I want people to accept me for what I am."

This cry of the sixties, which echoes on today, may seem to make sense. But unfortunately, the world accepts you for what it *sees* you to be. And most of what it sees is your clothes. Appropriate clothing is a mute persuader. It convinces people to trust you and your abilities. Psychologists tell us it takes just ninety seconds for another person to form an opinion of you. That's not a lot of time to make a first impression. And unfortunately, you don't always have the opportunity to make a second impression.

In his book, *Dress for Success*, John Molloy asserts that when you step into a room, even though no one has seen you before or knows you, it is possible to make ten decisions based on your appearance:

1. Economic level
2. Educational level
3. Trustworthiness
4. Social position
5. Level of sophistication
6. Economic heritage
7. Social heritage
8. Educational heritage
9. Your success
10. Your moral character

Further, he declares that people rarely alter their initial decisions about you. Actually, this is nothing new. Throughout history, most fashions were a symbol of belonging to a privileged social group. By imitating the dress of the privileged group, a person attempted to dissociate himself from his own social class and identify with a higher class.

Barbara Dickstern, collector of twentieth-century clothing for the Smithsonian Institute said, "Clothing, more than anything else— more than furniture, more than jewelry, clothing represents a person. No matter what the time frame, clothing is always a symbol of who you are. It tells your status, your role in life, your social position."

The distinctions in clothing and class are less obvious today, but the symbols are still there. Very subtle differences send the messages which Malloy lists.

Do you question the accuracy of this? Think a moment about watching a movie, a TV drama, a play. What gives you your first clue about the characters? Certainly the economic, social, educational, and even moral status of the characters are communicated to you before they speak, simply by the way they appear.

But, you say, that isn't fair in real life. You prefer to look past superficial appearance to the heart of the person. All right. Supposing your regular baby-sitter is not available and you must go to the hospital to visit your ailing mother. You call a sitter service which a trusted friend recommends. But when the sitter arrives, her hair is uncombed and oily, hanging in clumps over her face. Her clothes are early thrift store, somber-colored, and several sizes too large for her. The buttons on her sweater do not match. She wears very high-heeled strappy sandals and her purse is see-through plastic. Her eyes don't quite seem to focus, and there's an odd odor about her. Would you let her into your home and leave your children with her?

Everything you wear, including how you wear your hair, sends messages. Like it or not, it has been true since Adam and Eve.

Consider the fig leaf. When Adam and Eve covered themselves, weren't they sending a message? Weren't they signaling their shame and guilt? Until they ate of the tree of knowledge, they hadn't even known they were naked, much less felt embarrassment over it. God saw them and immediately received the message.

A number of women in the Bible understood the language of clothes. Esther dressed herself meticulously as she prepared to go before the king to ask his intervention in Haman's evil plot. Tamar programmed her father-in-law's response by taking off her widow's garments and covering herself with a veil. Just as she planned, he mistook her for a prostitute. And Naomi urged Ruth to bathe, use perfume, and put on a pretty garment before going to Boaz.

"PACKAGING" YOURSELF

In our Uniquely You seminars, I often liken clothing to packaging. Manufacturers, I point out, know that how they package a product profoundly affects how well it sells. They spend millions on attractive, eye-catching designs. I show the group a beautifully gift-wrapped box, and one covered with brown paper, tied with string.

"Which," I ask, "would you open first?"

The psychology of packaging embraces color appeal, silhouette or shape, and "product description."

Since clothes cover as much as 90 percent of your body, they are your packaging and provide most of the material with which people will judge you.

Sometimes, to illustrate this point, I bring a pretty, petite woman up from the audience and dress her in a huge, long, shapeless bright orange polyester jacket. Usually the group appreciates the example and dissolves in laughter. But recently, for the first time, a woman stalked out, muttering to no one in particular that the Lord loves us all and that's all that matters.

Of course, the Lord loves us all. But we are not he. In our humanness, we do make judgments—and so does everyone else. They see your packaging long before they notice the wonderful woman inside. Before you open your mouth, your clothes start talking for you.

It stands to reason, then, that if you want to be successful—whether you define success as a better job or being a more effective witness to others—you'll "package" yourself to say what you want to say to those who are important to you.

Does this sound manipulative to you? It seems to me that since we must wear *something*, it's only good sense to choose "something" which will help others form positive opinions about your honesty, your background, your friendliness, and your intent.

Packaging is the key to "impression management," and it works.

THE MESSAGE OF YOUR APPEARANCE

Let's look at some of the messages our appearance can transmit. Come with me into a shopping center, to watch the passing parade. Here comes a woman who is dressed in a putty color; she has light, uncombed hair and pale skin. Nothing relieves the monochrome. She's *blah*. Further, the cut of her blouse and pants emphasizes her very generously proportioned lower half. The message? "Don't bother with me. I don't care about myself, and you probably wouldn't be interested in me either."

Behind her jiggles a voluptuous teenager. No bra, very brief knit top with shoulder straps, shorts too short to cover her derriere. A young man on a nearby bench sums it up succinctly. "She's lookin' for it!" he mutters.

Now we see a graying woman in her late forties. She's a bit overweight, but her suit is of a classic cut, the A-line skirt flattering to her hips. The color, a sapphire blue, makes her skin glow, her eyes look deeply blue; her graying hair glistens. Here's a woman who is expressing in her dress how she cares about herself. You're drawn to her, feel you'd like to know her.

Women seem naturally more concerned with relationships than with external appearances, and they tend to forget how very visual men are by nature. According to Dr. Joyce Brothers, "The average man makes up his mind in seven short seconds whether or not he wants to know a woman better." You don't have much time to make your impression!

Listen to the preoccupation with the visual in the biblical Song of Solomon: "I compare you, my love, to a mare of Pharaoh's chariots, your cheeks are comely with ornaments, your neck with strings of jewels." Or, "Behold, you are beautiful, my love. . . . Your eyes are doves behind your veil."

We need to remember this, especially if we are dressing for our husbands. Men may receive messages we never intended when we decided to buy that bikini or that dress with the plunging neckline.

Or, consider the woman who couldn't understand why the men in her office wouldn't take her seriously. She puzzled over this while wearing a little-girl dress with ruffles and an Orphan Annie hair style.

And what about your appearance at home? How you present yourself affects how your family reacts to you. As your husband leaves in the morning for a working world populated with many women, how does he remember you? In a bathrobe, with no makeup? In jeans and your adolescent son's outgrown shirt? Or as a single person, how do you look when you answer the door for an unexpected caller?

Children, too, are far more observant than we sometimes realize. How we dress tells them what we feel about ourselves, and also how we feel about them. If we are not "together" looking, we give off subtle vibes of confusion, while telling children they're not important enough to "dress" for.

A neighbor admits that, when in haste she pulls her hair back in a ponytail, her young child disapprovingly pulls it apart. Another says her teenage sons treat her with much more consideration when she dons a simple cotton skirt and a soft blouse than when she settles for cutoffs and a T-shirt.

Your appearance profoundly affects the way you're treated by others outside the home, too, in a social gathering, in a restaurant, or in a store.

One of my consultants was shopping recently in a department store, and she looked so radiant, so put-together that the clerk couldn't believe the three children she had piled into the stroller were all hers. The salesperson couldn't do enough to help her.

Can we say that clothing doesn't matter?

If you're not sure what messages your own clothing is giving, make it a point to watch for the responses you get from others. Often, they reflect back your own signals. If, for instance, you're told, "Now, don't bother your pretty little head over this," or asked, "Would this be too much for you to handle?" perhaps a very youthful or frivolous appearance is casting doubts on your competence.

A "Who cares?" response from your teenager might also reflect your own "Who cares?" attitude about your appearance at home.

I think you'll be amazed if you try testing your clothes and making notes on the feedback you receive.

For not only does your clothing give off signals; it also tends to be self-fulfilling. The teenager who appears to be "lookin' for it" will probably "get it." And the tragedy is, she may not understand why. The woman who *looks* colorless and apologetic, *is*.

The more unattractive you feel, the more you tend to withdraw. And as others react negatively or ignore you, you retreat more and more.

Conversely, when you dress becomingly, there often is a mirror effect. As you feel positive about the way you look, you have more confidence and begin reaching out.

Nowhere is this more apparent than in Uniquely You's work with delinquents. These young women are down on themselves, down on the world. But when they learn to wear their most becoming colors, discover the lines and designs in clothing which flatter them most (and eliminate the unflattering), they perceive themselves and the rest of the world quite differently. Destructive attitudes and behavior diminish. They have hope.

My files are full of letters which express similar changes in women's lives. Nothing is more gratifying to me.

Today, won't you honestly consider what message your appearance sends to the world? Do you radiate confidence? Are you saying, "I am filled with God's harmony, peace, hope, and love"? Or is your message, "I'm not quite sure. Ask me some other time."

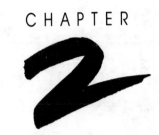

BEAUTY IS PERSPECTIVE

HOW DOES GOD SEE YOU?

Do you ever feel really down on yourself, convinced that you're inadequate as a daughter or a mother, a wife, a friend, an employee, a manager, a woman, a *person?*

This is the plight of most women I meet: they feel they have to be perfect. Their biggest life challenge is to overcome a sense of not being acceptable.

Let me create a "feeling picture" of what it's like to be accepted. It's like a big, warm *hug*, which surrounds you with a sense of being secure, protected, wanted, loved, cherished.

This is a picture of how God accepts us, his children.

A friend told me of a wonderfully revealing experience with her father which parallels our relationship with our heavenly Father.

She admitted that she felt she had never done enough for her father, particularly in recent years after her mother died and her dad became confined to a wheelchair. He lived 1,500 miles away and would not move closer to my friend. So she visited him twice a year.

In the meantime, her brother-in-law, Jim, who lived near her father, was an enormous help to him. He ran errands, cooked dinner every Sunday, and stopped by frequently. So one summer, when Jim was away on vacation, my friend went to visit her father.

The second evening, her father suddenly turned to her and began berating Jim, terming him "selfish," adding, "He just couldn't wait to get out of town."

Fully aware of how unselfishly Jim cared for her father, she responded angrily, "What are you saying, Dad, that Jim shouldn't take a vacation—that he should stay here with you?"

Her father glared at her and shouted, "I don't want to fight about this!"

"I don't either, Dad," she said, tears welling up in her eyes.

They sat silent for a moment. Then she said, "Dad, I understand that you miss Jim, but when you tell me he doesn't do enough for you, I feel dreadful. You see, I know how much more he does for you than I do, and I know I don't do *nearly* enough."

"That's different," her father snapped. "I've never felt that you owe me anything. I don't expect you to repay me for anything I've done for you. You are mine, and I love you very, very much."

Afterward, my friend marveled at her father's attitude. How could he overlook her selfishness, her inadequacies? His love was undemanding. It did not depend upon what she did or did not do. It was total. It was unconditional.

It was, indeed, a reflection of her heavenly Father's perspective of her!

A woman recently told me, "I could never be a Christian, because I could never do all those things."

"Do what things?" I asked.

She hesitated. Then, "Well, you know—be perfect, like Jesus."

I reminded her of the bumper sticker, "Christians aren't perfect; just forgiven."

Do you remember the kinds of people Jesus chose to spend time with? Tax collectors, who were considerd by many only slightly more desirable company than lepers. Prostitutes. Remember the woman at the well? Remember Mary Magdalene? And remember who God selected to carry the news of Jesus' resurrection? That's right: Mary Magdalene.

Matthew, Mark, and Luke all quote Jesus, replying to those who criticized the company he kept: "It is not the healthy who need a doctor, but the sick. . . . I have not come to call the righteous. . . ."

But if we are not righteous, how do we become acceptable in God's eyes? By depending on Jesus who made us right with God when he offered for all time, one sacrifice for our sins. By his one sacrifice he has made us perfect forever (Hebrews 10:12, 14).

So you see, as Peter Gillquist says, God does not say, "I love you if . . ." but "I love you." Period!

This is why God could look at Mary Magdalene and say, "I don't care what you used to be; I care that you're believing in me."

He is saying to each of us, "I don't care that you're _____ .

[You fill in the blank!] I care that you're believing me."

Moreover, God's love for us is a strong, enduring love. Listen to Paul's description: "Neither death nor life, neither angels nor demons, neither the present nor the future, nor any powers, neither height nor depth, nor anything else in all creation, will be able to separate us from the love of God that is in Christ Jesus our Lord" (Romans 8:38, 39).

Personal worth, then, is God's gift to us. We don't earn it like Brownie points, and we can't win it through our performance.

It took me a long, long time to realize this. There were years when I was overwhelmed with the pressure to perform. I took Christian tracts to the beach. I felt guilty if I didn't witness to the stranger next to me on an airplane, or if I hadn't spent at least an hour in devotions. I thought, like my friend, that I could never do enough for my Father.

Of course, I still want to do what is pleasing to him, but this desire is my response to our love relationship; I no longer feel burdened by a long list of "gottas." In fact, only when I understood how completely acceptable I am to God, just as I am, did I begin to have the freedom to reach out and to be of value to others.

Moreover, one of the greatest benefits of knowing that God loves and accepts us is that *we* can risk looking honestly at *ourselves*, and learning to accept ourselves, just as we are.

TAKING AN HONEST LOOK AT YOUR BODY: FEARFULLY AND WONDERFULLY MADE

I have *never* met a woman who liked everything about her appearance. We are *so* critical of ourselves! Even actress Sophia Loren, I read recently, is not totally happy with her looks. In an interview with *Family Weekly* she said, "Personally, I find my shoulders too broad, my hips too narrow, my eyes something less than remarkable...."

I personally do not like my small head or my knock knees. (As a youngster, I wondered why, when I stretched my legs out in the bathtub, my knees didn't point up. I drew faces on my knees, and they smiled at each other!)

And here's a dialogue I heard recently outside a department store dressing room.

"I think," said the well-rounded woman gazing at herself in a mirror, "that I look exactly like a Bartlett pear in this bathing suit."

"Don't complain," responded a painfully thin woman who'd just

THE A-SHAPE

Narrow shoulders

Possibly a small bustline

Round, broader hips

If the lines are well rounded, this could be your basic pear shape. This body type carries the weight in the hips.

THE H-V SHAPE

Essentially straight up and down; the "athletic" build (H-shape)

Broader at the shoulders (V-shape)

Slim or no hips

Flat derriere

This shape tends to gain weight in the middle.

T-SHAPE

Generally slender form

"T" is in the thighs; body widest across thighs

This body shape tends to accumulate weight at the cross of the "T" and through the legs.

THE X-SHAPE

Shoulders and hips are about equal in width, with smaller waistline. Depending upon how much of you there is, this could be the Renoir or hour-glass shape. The X generally gains weight all over the body.

emerged for a full-length view of herself. "I look like an eleven-year-old boy in this suit."

"I should be so lucky!" came a voice from a nearby cubicle.

There's nothing like trying on bathing suits to bring that moment of truth. We *are* "fearfully and wonderfully made." And sometimes we wonder about the "wonderfully"!

But made by whom? By God! We are his own design. Who, then, are we to criticize his handiwork?

Instead, let's look realistically at how we are created. We must understand that less than 10 percent of all women have so-called "perfect" shapes. That makes the rest of us *normal.* (And remember, what is considered perfect in the United States is very different from what's considered perfect in other parts of the world. In some cultures, for instance, the large frame is beautiful.) Further, since 90 percent of us are so-called "imperfect," what we are is certainly what God meant us to be.

So let's learn what we have to work with, admit it, and accept it.

"Not now," you say.

Yes, now.

"After I lose those pounds. After that aerobic dancing class."

No, now. You can be beautiful now, no matter what you weigh, no matter how old you are, no matter how many or how great your so-called flaws. (And who says they're flaws? That 1 percent minority?)

We need to understand our body shape to know what clothing will most flatter us, and to avoid expensive mistakes in our shopping. Otherwise, what we buy will always be a guess.

So what is your basic body shape? If you have trouble defining it, it might help you to lightly outline the reflection of your body in a full-length mirror with a sliver of soap. Now step back. What do you have?

Pictured in the middle on the next page is that rarity, the perfectly proportioned body, sometimes termed the $2.98 body, because this person can wear inexpensive off-the-rack clothes and look great in them.

If you're not sure how you shape up, let's get more specific and look at various measurements to see how they relate to your height and bone structure. Here are some "ideal" measurements for various heights. They will help you determine which of your "parts" are relatively large, relatively small, or "perfect."

Remember, very few ever achieve the so-called ideal!

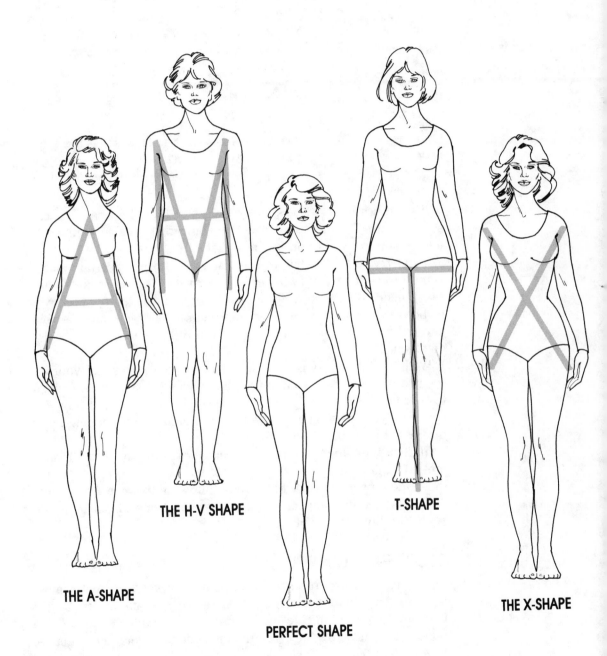

THE H-V SHAPE

T-SHAPE

THE A-SHAPE

PERFECT SHAPE

THE X-SHAPE

BASIC MEASUREMENT GAUGE	SHORT	AVERAGE	MEDIUM TALL	TALL
	Under 5'4"	5'4½"– 5'6½"	5'7"–5'9"	Over 5'9"
Normal wrist	5½"–6"	5¾"–6½"	6"–7"	6½"–7½"
Bust	32–33	34–35	35–37	38–39
Waist	22–23	23–25	25–27	28–29
Hip	32–33	34–35	35–37	38–39
Upper thigh	18½	19	19½	20
Calf	12½	13	13½	14
Ankle	7½	8	8½	9
Upper arm	8½	9	9½	10

It's important to understand your figure type, because you can starve yourself or eat and eat, but you won't change your basic figure. You are what you are, and that's it!

Don't try to fight what you are. It is OK to be a certain size. I want to repeat that. *It is OK to be a certain size.* I find that women really need to hear this, because we are so besieged by directives to be *thin.* I have had women approach me in tears after a class and tell me, "No one ever told me before that it's OK to be a size eighteen."

Well, it is! Accept what you are. Then learn to dress for yourself today, to be the best you can be. Even when I work with weight-loss groups, I encourage acceptance of the body as it is now, because as you dress slimmer, you look slimmer and become more interested in losing weight.

In deciding which clothes you wear most effectively, it's important to understand your proportions. Few of us, of course, have those ideal proportions which would allow us to wear almost anything. But we can appear to be well proportioned by using compensating lines in our clothing.

DISCOVERING YOUR FIGURE TYPE

To determine your proportions, stand in your stocking feet against a door or wall and ask a friend to make tiny pencil marks (or use masking tape) to indicate just where each shoulder bone and hip bone is located. Now, measure the distances between these marks. In the ideal figure, the shoulders are an inch wider than the hips, to allow clothing to fall loosely over the hips from the shoulders.

If you find that your hips are more than an inch wider than your shoulders, you know that you are more A-shaped. If your shoulders are more than an inch wider than your hips, you are V-shaped. If they are equal, you are either X-shaped or H-shaped, depending upon whether or not your waist is distinctly narrower than your shoulders and hips.

Next, let's see if you're long- or short-legged, long- or short-waisted. Mark your height on the door or wall. Then, lift your knee and notice where your thigh bends from your torso. Make a mark at this point. Measure both marks from the floor. If your legs are half of your height, you have average length legs. If you're more than an inch "off" either way, you may want to compensate in your dress, though a slightly longer-legged look can be very attractive.

Now, mark the door or wall at your armpit and at your waist. Ideally, the waist lies halfway between your armpit and the joint where the thigh joins the torso. If your measurement varies more than an inch, you are either short-waisted or long-waisted.

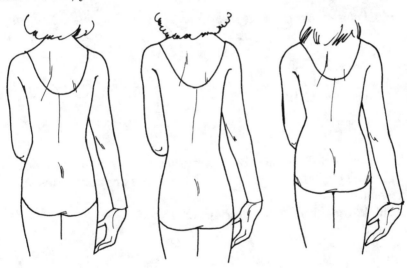

To determine your arm length, let your arms hang at your sides. Again, lift your knee and notice where your thigh bends from your hips. If the first knuckle of your thumb aligns with the crotch, and if your elbow is even with your waist, your arms are average length.

You should also know whether your head is large or small, since a small head makes you look taller, while a large head shortens. So, turn sideways to the wall, and have someone make a mark just below your chin. Now measure the distance from the top of your head to beneath your chin. If it is one-eighth the length of your entire body, your head is well proportioned to your body. If it's smaller and you are tall, you may want to compensate with a more bouffant hair style, although models love a small-headed look. If it's larger and you are short, keep your hair sleekly trimmed.

Finally, let's determine whether your neck is long or short. Looking straight ahead, place your hand horizontally just beneath your chin with your palm against your throat, fingers together. If you can touch your collar bone with your little finger without spreading your other fingers, you have a short neck. If you must expand your fingers till there's a half-inch between, your neck is medium long. If you must spread your fingers still further to touch your collar bone, you have a long neck.

Now you're ready to fill in your figure line analysis on page 30. (Be sure to note whether your waist is high or low, narrow or thick.)

Now, how about your shoulders: wide or narrow? Also, note your shoulders. Are they:

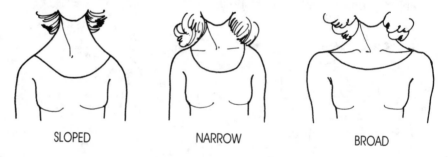

SLOPED   NARROW   BROAD

Is your neck long or short? Arms, heavy or thin? Long or short? Legs, long or short, thick or thin? Bust, large or small? Hips, ample or small?

Think, too, about your derriere or buttocks.
Are they:

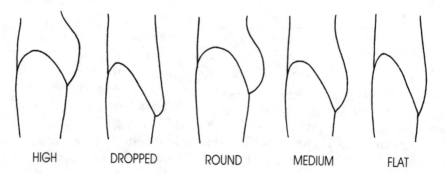

HIGH   DROPPED   ROUND   MEDIUM   FLAT

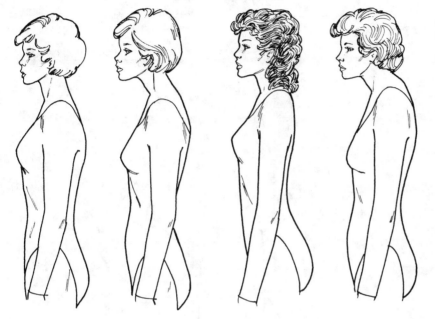

And how about your posture or carriage? Do you carry your head thrust forward?

Or do you have a swayback you should consider?

Or perhaps a dowager's hump?

Consider, too, the shape of your face. With your hair pulled back, what is its basic geometric shape? Round? Oval? Square? Rectangular? Triangular? A combination, such as an oval with a square jaw? (You'll find drawings of the various face shapes on p. 126 of chapter 6.)

Now you know what you're working with. Are you feeling a little discouraged? Don't be. This is the beginning of learning how you can best enhance your basic figure shape and proportions. The key lies in understanding that the eye sees lines in a certain way, and we can use this to our advantage. It's called optical illusion. Basically, the eye follows lines until they are broken or turned in another direction.

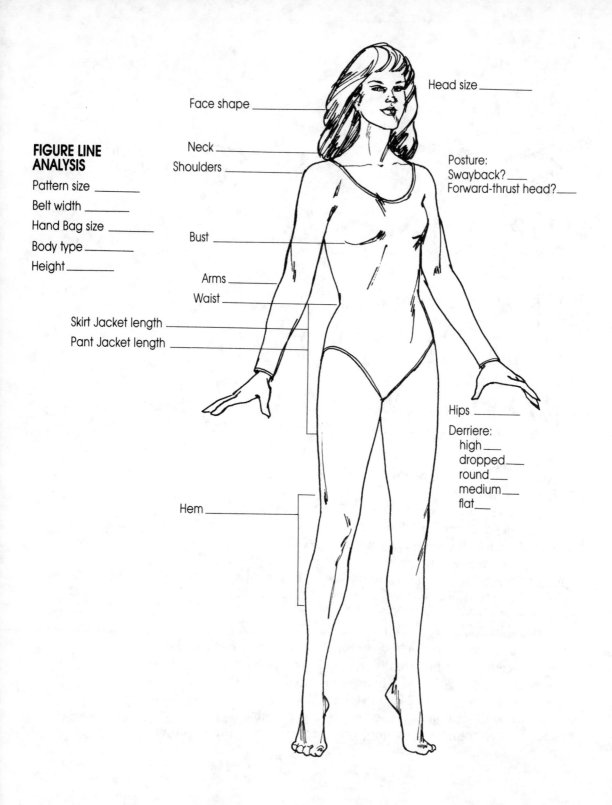

Head size _____

Face shape _____

Posture:
Swayback? _____
Forward-thrust head? _____

FIGURE LINE ANALYSIS

Neck _____
Shoulders _____

Pattern size _____
Belt width _____
Hand Bag size _____
Body type _____
Height _____

Bust _____

Arms _____
Waist _____

Skirt Jacket length _____
Pant Jacket length _____

Hips _____

Derriere:
high _____
dropped _____
round _____
medium _____
flat _____

Hem _____

Horizontals. Horizontal lines, of course, emphasize width, because they keep the eye moving from side to side, rather than up and down.

Like this:

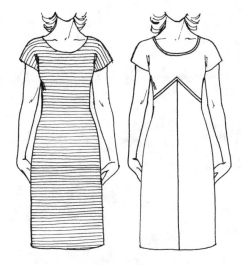

Note how these crossways lines shorten, broaden, and tend to round the body.
Wide skirt panels do the same thing!

And this:

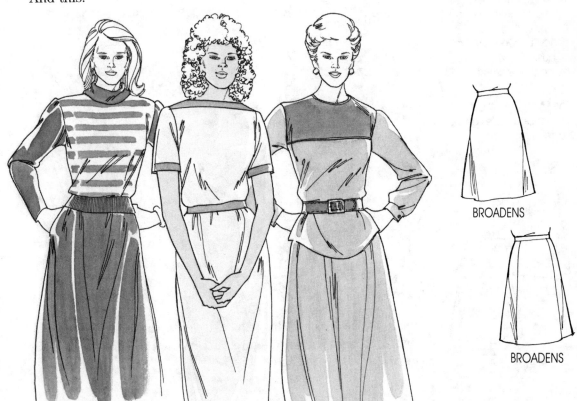

BROADENS

BROADENS

Verticals. Vertical lines in detailing, patterns, or silhouette, lead the eye up and down. They make you appear taller and slimmer.

Like this:

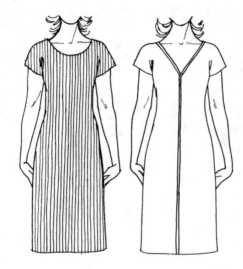

The princess line adds height. (For the most slimming effect, the center panel should be no wider than the space between crowns of bust, unless broken by center seam or placket.)

The "Magic Y" makes you appear taller and slimmer.

And this:

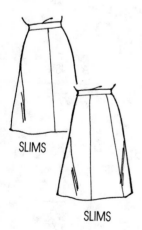

SLIMS

SLIMS

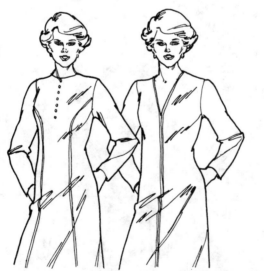

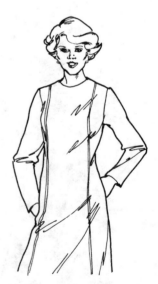

However, two vertical lines placed far apart will definitely add weight and shorten your figure. Note how the three wide panels draw the eye *across* the body.

Yet these vertical seams are slimming.

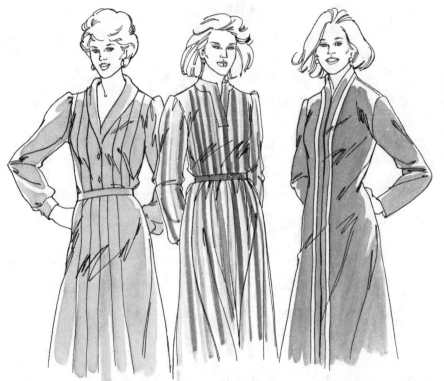

Diagonals. Diagonal lines may either broaden or lengthen, depending upon the angle and the length of the line. A short diagonal leads the eye sideways and gives the impression of width. A longer diagonal gives a narrower impression and leads the eye more downward than across. Diagonals are softer and more subtle than verticals and horizontals, and can be extremely effective.

Curves. Curved lines lead the eye in the same manner as straight lines, but are much less obvious. In draping, seaming, or edges, they give a softer, more feminine look, since they emphasize the curves of the body. (See illustration on following page.)

Illusion of Size. In addition, if the figure is surrounded by items which are large, it appears smaller. If it's surrounded by small things, it appears larger. The center circles in this illustration are actually the same size.

How does this apply to our appearance? I have a small face and

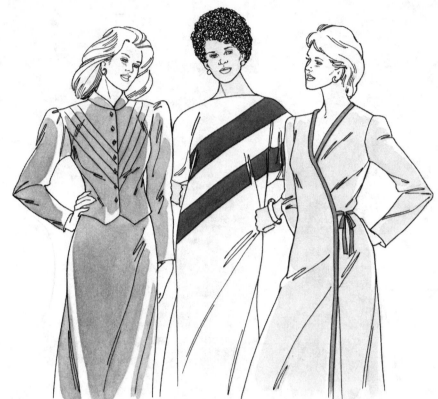

must wear small earrings to make my face look bigger. Yet I recently met a woman who owned an antique jewelry store, who insisted upon wearing huge earrings to display her wares. With her tiny face, she was completely out of balance.

We see the same principle in clothing. Small bows at the neck (and small gold chains) tend to broaden the shoulders. Larger bows (and necklaces) make the shoulders appear smaller and narrower.

Does this help you to see why a tent dress and an oversize purse can dwarf a small woman, but help a large woman appear smaller? By the same token, a tiny print can give the illusion of decreased size to a generously proportioned woman, while it may make a tiny woman look more substantial.

Patterns in fabrics may be used both to create lines (vertical, horizontal, or diagonal) and to give illusions of size, width, slimness, and balance. (If they're too "busy," however, they're distracting. People see the garment before they see you.)

Another often-neglected factor in the illusion of size and shape is the texture of a fabric. Material which is bulky or heavy or coarse,

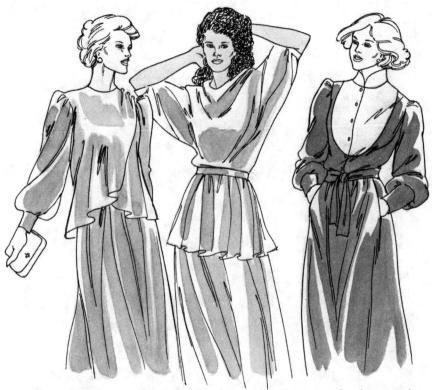

such as tweed, wool, or wide-wale corduroy, gives the impression of added physical dimension and appears to add pounds to your body—great for the tall and thin.

Stiff fabric, such as taffeta, stands away from the body and can hide some imperfections and irregularities. It's good on average-to-tall figures with average or slender bodies. The tiny and large should avoid it.

Shiny fabrics, such as satin and polished cotton, reflect light and intensify the color, making the wearer appear larger. Fabrics such as plush, velvet, velour, and corduroy both reflect and absorb light and are fine for the slender, not for the generously proportioned.

However, dull textures absorb light and do not enlarge the figure. Challis, cotton knit, gabardine, suede cloth, and fine, light woolens are suitable for most body types.

Sheer or transparent fabrics are usually layered or ruffled and thus add weight. Silk chiffon is an exception.

Transparent and clingy fabrics reveal the figure—just how much of it you have, whether it's too much, too little, or just right. For

Now, let's see how the principles of line and proportion can be applied to the different body types.

FIGURE TYPE A

The goal in the silhouette is to balance the broad beam by widening the shoulders. (See p. 45 for specific ideas on working with narrow shoulders and p. 56 for suggestions on broad hips.) Stay away from lines which call attention to hips.

FIGURE TYPE H

Strive to create the illusion of an hourglass shape to look more like the rounded X. Avoid lines which are too boxy or too skimpy.

FIGURE TYPE V

Work toward adding roundness and to give the illusion of the hourglass. Widen the hips to balance the shoulders. (See p. 46 for specifics on broad shoulders and p. 57 for ideas on dealing with narrow hips.) Avoid skimpy clothes or anything which further broadens the shoulder.

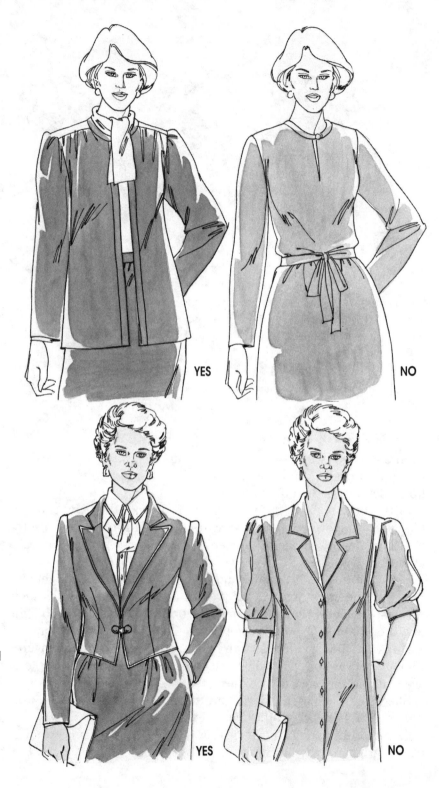

YES

NO

YES

NO

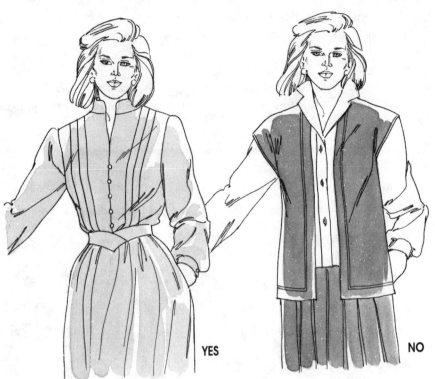

FIGURE TYPE X

If you're of average weight, emphasize what you are: a graceful hourglass. Avoid cluttering the frame with too much or hiding its charms with boxy lines.

LARGE FRAME X FIGURE TYPE

If you're an overweight X, work toward an H-shape silhouette. Avoid tight-fitting garments and fluffy excesses of material.

YES

NO

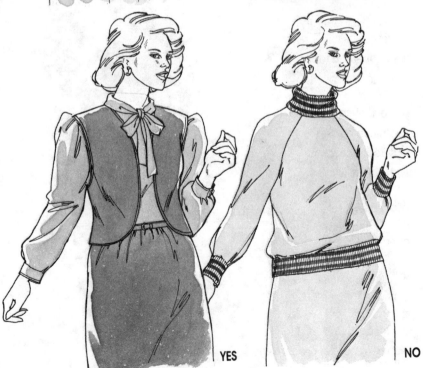

FIGURE TYPE T

Emphasize the top half of the silhouette in order to balance the width at the thighs. Work toward an H-shape, avoiding anything which adds bulk or calls attention to the lower hip or upper thigh.

YES

NO

No to:

Clinging fabrics or tight garments

Small-scale collars, buttons, accessories

Three-quarter sleeves (make arms look longer)

"Little-girl" dresses

Empire lines

Vertical stripes and other vertical effects

Very short hair

Short skirts

Boleros

Severely tailored lines

Shifts, with no horizontal lines

Flat heels

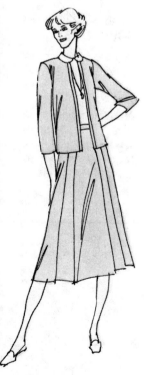

nightgowns, fine; office blouses, no.

Probably you already have a good sense of which fabric textures are right for you. But for some women, this is a revelation. I remember one 4'8" woman who wore a wool fleece jacket and wide-wale corduroy skirt—and managed to look like a toadstool. And an overweight woman does herself no favor in choosing a large plaid suit.

Now, let's look at specific needs.

If you're tall and would like to look shorter: *Yes* to:

The layered look

Large, flaring sleeves

Ponchos

Long jackets

Bulky fabrics

Horizontal lines, especially toward bottom of dress or skirt

Three-quarter-length jackets

Bold patterned fabrics

Outfits in contrasting colors

Large-scale accessories

Two-piece dresses

Textured fabrics

Two vertical lines, placed far apart

Wider belts

Capes and cape effects

Suits and dresses with soft lines

Gathered or pleated skirts

Lighter colors

High heels (better proportion)

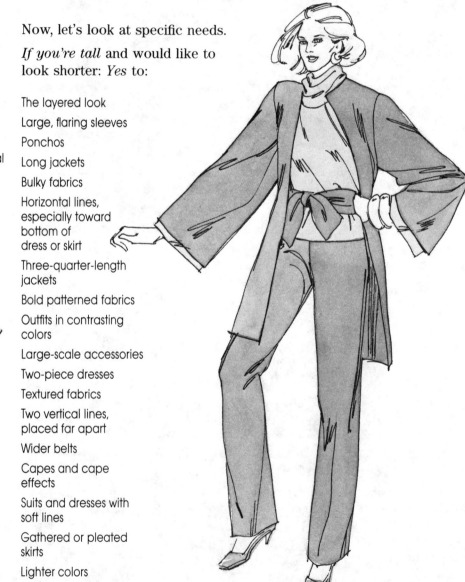

If you're short and would like to look taller:
Yes to:

Simplicity and long-lined design

Hair swept up from face

One color, or a very gentle contrast of colors

Fitted coats, vests, short jackets

Vertical neckline; low, open neckline

Line of vertical buttons

Cuffless sleeves; long or 3/4 sleeves

Slim or slightly flared skirts

Horizontal line high on body, such as an empire waist

Boleros

Small patterns; smooth fabrics

Hem not too long or short

Princess lines

Hosiery and shoe matched to color of hem

Pumps

Unbroken lines

Shoulder-to-hemline seams

Jump suits

Small scale accessories; thin chains

Straight-leg pants

Chanel jacket

Narrow belts, same color as dress

Smooth fabrics

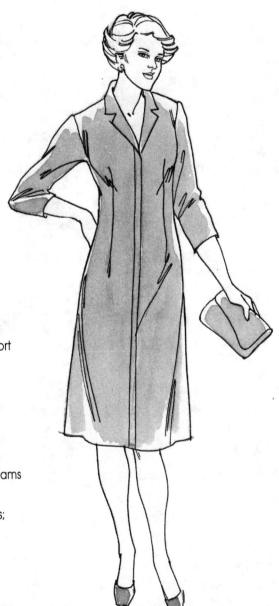

No to:

Lines in hair and hat which turn down

Billowing skirts

Heavy fabrics

Horizontal lines or construction

Contrasting bold colors

Being too cute: ruffles, puffed sleeves

Large patterns

Out-of-scale bag

Loose, draped garments

Long skirts (or too-short skirts)

Heavy boots

Pegged-leg pants

Frills and fancy lace

More than three colors

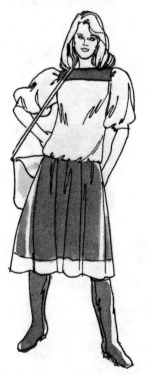

No to:

Hair that's longer than shoulder length or full

Horizontal scarf at neck

Sleeveless tops

Bare midriffs

Clingy fabrics

Clothes which are tight

Shorts or short skirts

Heavy tweeds, bulky knits, big furs

Splashy figures or prints

Caftans

Shiny, lustrous fabrics, rigid fabrics

Fitted, frilly, fussy, or stretchy garments

Dainty jewelry

Ankle straps

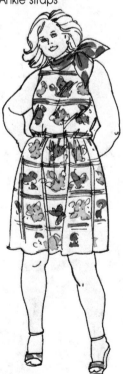

If you're average height:

Lucky you! Seldom do you need alterations, and shopping is easier. What may overpower the short girl or be lost on the tall girl will probably look great on you.

If you'd like to look slimmer:

Yes to:

V-necklines

Necklines that point eye toward face

Long necklaces

Full length or three-quarter sleeves

Jackets without lapels; long jackets covering derriere

Loosely shaped garments; no waist emphasis

Muted colors; subdued prints

Two vertical lines placed close together; vertical pinstripes

Pants with overblouse

Sheer wools, crepe; medium-weight fabrics

Smooth or matte finish fabrics

Medium plaids, checks

Front-wrap skirts

The "magic Y"

Long, straight coat

Skirts with slight flare

Skirts with narrow-paneled gores

Darker colors in unbroken line

Diagonal lines at bust

Pumps in proportion to body

Solid colors in darker tones

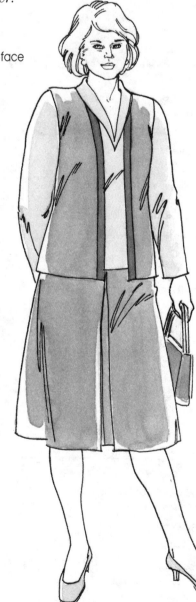

If you feel you're too thin:
Yes to:

Blousy dresses, tops

Full-cut bodices

Long, full sleeves

Gentle, soft lines

Full or gathered skirts

Soft cowl necklines

Shirtwaist dresses with long sleeves

Pantsuits

Fabrics which are soft and full, giving illusion of more shape

Soft, rounded accessories

Light or bright tights

Contrasting belts

Chokers and dickeys

Light colors

The layered look

Contrasting colors

Fabrics which add bulk, fullness

Plaids, checks, and patterns

Textured stockings

Boots

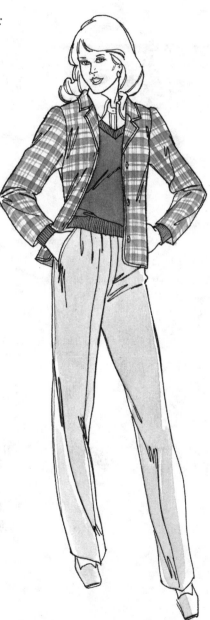

No to:

V-necks

Long diagonal lines

Short sleeves

Clingy or bare garments

Tubular dresses

Garments without belts

Princess lines

Dark, one-color outfits

Narrow skirts

Skirts which are too long (or too short, skimpy)

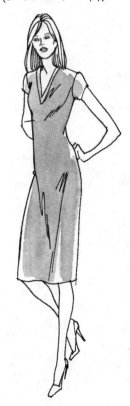

Next, let's deal with particular parts of this wonderful, unique body God gave you, and learn how to accentuate or minimize them. We'll start at the top and work down.

If you have a round or square face:

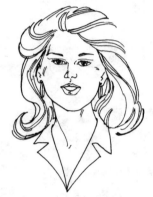 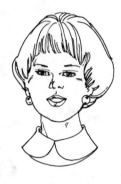

Yes to:

Necklines which contrast to the shape of your face

Long necklaces

V-shaped, collarless necklines

Longer hair

Cardigan jacket

No to:

Necklines which repeat the lines of your face (Round face should not wear round neckline; square face should avoid square).

Chanel jacket

If you have a long face:

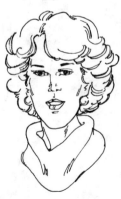 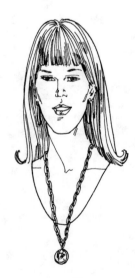

Yes to:

Necklines and jewelry which cut
the long line

Bow necks, turtlenecks

Soft gathers, ruffles at neck

Chanel jacket

No to:

Long necklaces

V-necks and collarless tops

Long hair

Cardigan

If you have a double chin:

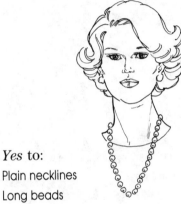 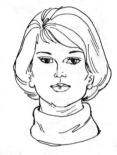

Yes to:

Plain necklines

Long beads

Anything which centers attention
on your hair and eyes

No to:

Turtlenecks

Choker necklaces

If you'd like to minimize age lines:

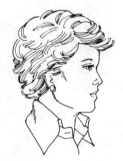 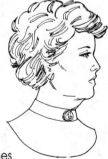

Yes to:

Open, high-standing
collar

Wide turtleneck or cowl

Soft necklines: ruffles

No to:

Scoop necklines

High turtlenecks

Choker necklaces

High round or jewel neck

Tightly wrapped scarves

If you have a long neck:

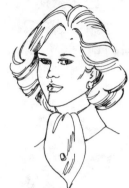
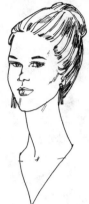

Yes to:

Hairstyles which cover
nape of neck

Turtlenecks, cowl necks, high necks

Boat necks

Filling in with scarves, chokers

Round earrings

One-shouldered evening dresses

Oxford collars

Mandarin collars

Drawstring ruffle necks

Hats with downward lines

No to:

Upswept hairstyles

Very short hair

Peter Pan collars

Scoop necks

Square necks

V-necks, deep-plunging necklines

Dolman sleeves

Cardigan jackets

Long pendants, dangling earrings

Strapless gowns

*If your neck is
very short:*

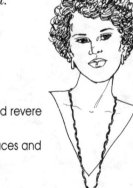
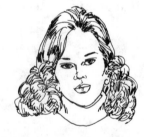

Yes to:

Long pointed revere
collars

Long necklaces and
pendants

V-necks

Tapered hair styles

Lighter colors at neck

Cardigan jackets

No to:

Classic T-shirt

Long hair

Bulky scarves or bows under chin

Turtleneck

Mandarin or Peter Pan collars

Jewel necks

If your head is set forward, or you have a *dowager's hump:*

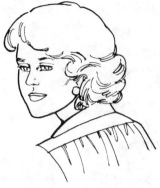 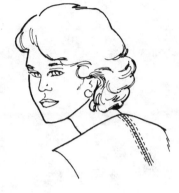

Yes to:

Hair with fullness at back

Collars which stand away from the
back of the neck

Scarves which help fill in back of neck

Gathered yoke across shoulders

No to:

Drop shoulders

Jewel necklines

Anything clingy or formfitting

Back zippers at neck

If you have narrow and/or sloping shoulders:

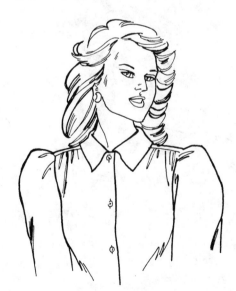 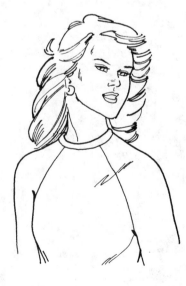

Yes to:

Padded shoulders
Heavy fabrics
Small collars
Shirts with set-in sleeves
Puffed sleeves
Moving shoulder seams out
Drop shoulders
Horizontal yokes
Fly-front jacket
Slender waist and hiplines
V-necks
Boat necks
Smooth, short-hair furs
Double-breasted jackets
Boxy jackets
Boleros
Halter tops
Cap Sleeves

No to:

Large coats and jackets
Turtlenecks
Raglan sleeves
Large lapels
Dresses with droopy, off-shoulder sleeves
Sleeveless tops
Dolman sleeves
Tight waists or jackets
Full skirts
Long, tight sleeves

If you have broad shoulders:

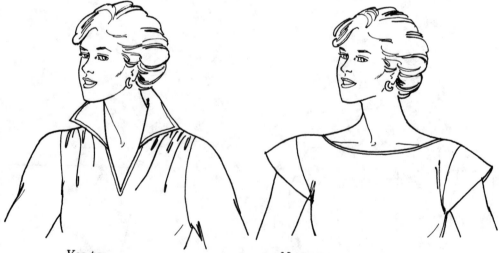

Yes to:

Raglan sleeves
Large collars

No to:

Puffed sleeves
Padded shoulders

Dolman sleeves

Shoulder lines one inch inside your natural shoulder line

V-necks

Vests

Kimono blouse

Narrow lapels

Unconstructed shirts and jackets with easy shoulder lines

Shoulders without a defined line

Cap sleeves

Boat necks

Broad horizontal patterns or stripes

Strapless gowns

V-neck with short sleeves

Shoulder trim, accent, or color

Small collars

High necklines

Drop shoulders

If you have thin arms:

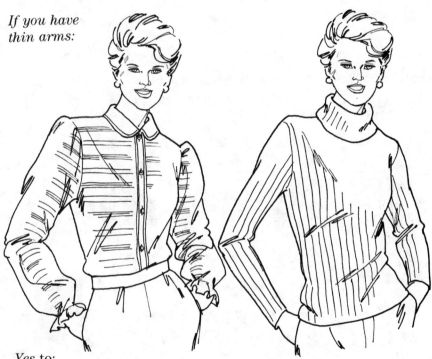

Yes to:

Sleeves that are wide, full above elbow

Loose-fitting sleeves

Draped or bulky sleeves, fitted at wrists

Horizontal lines in sleeves

Elbow-length or bracelet-length sleeves with cuffs

No to:

Tight sleeves (unless bulky fabric, or textured)

Turtlenecks

Cap sleeves

Sleeveless garments

Strapless gowns

If you have long arms:

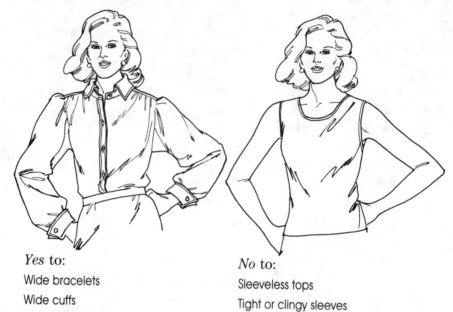

Yes to:

Wide bracelets

Wide cuffs

Fuller sleeves

Contrasting gloves

No to:

Sleeveless tops

Tight or clingy sleeves

Cap sleeves

*If you have
heavy arms:*

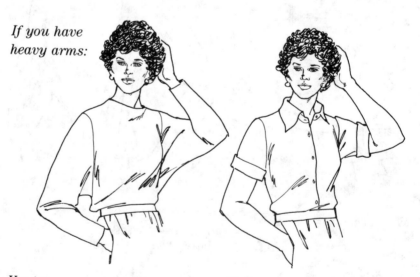

Yes to:

Raglan, dolman, or kimono sleeves

Wide armhole cuts

Long, cuffless, unbroken sleeve line

No to:

Tight or puffed sleeves

Clingy fabrics

Sleeveless or very short-sleeved styles

If your hands show aging:
Yes to:

Ruffles

Simple jewelry

Medium nails, neutral polish

Hand makeup (hides veins, "age" spots)

No to:

Three-quarter sleeves

Attention-getting jewelry

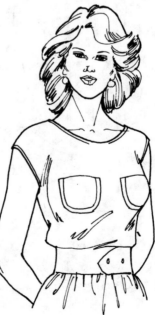
If your fingers are very long/bony:
Yes to:

Ruffles

Neutral to soft-colored nail polish

Larger rings

Fuller sleeves

No to:

Three-quarter sleeves

If your fingers are short, fat:
Yes to:

Long, slim sleeves

Neutral polish and longer nails

Cuffless sleeves

No to:

Horizontal cuffs, bracelets

Three-quarter sleeves

Bulky jewelry

Slim-banded rings

Turtlenecks

*If you have
a full bust:*

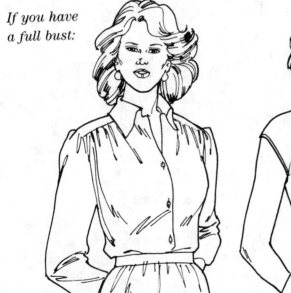

Yes to:

V-necks

Open collars

Silk shirts

Loose tops (if not too full)

Stand-up shawl collar jacket

One-button blazer

Dark colors on top, lighter on bottom

Diagonal lines

Minimizer bra

Center button shirts

No to:

Stiff fabrics

Fabrics that reveal bra lines

Lightweight or clinging fabrics

Tube tops

Dolman sleeves

Tight knits

Tight blouses

Patch pockets on shirts or dresses

Princess styling

Roll-up sleeves

If you have a short torso or waist:

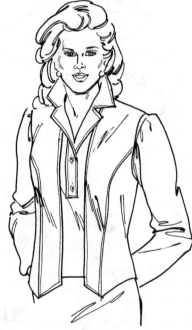 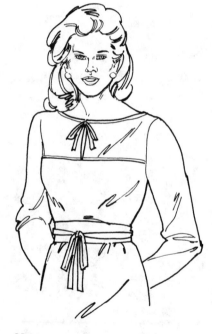

Yes to:

V-necks

Loose layers

Longer, open vests

Longer sweaters with pants, slim skirts

Outfits of one color or close tones

No to:

Bare midriff

Dresses that call attention to waist

Waist-defining separates

High waistbands on trousers

Tight T-shirts

No-waist dress

Unfitted jackets

Overblouses

Jacket and tunic lengths falling to pant inseam, or just above

Slacks that ride low on natural waist (hiphuggers, low-rise jeans)

Sweaters worn out over slacks, skirts

Blouson style dress or blouse

Horizontal bodice details

Wide belts

Very short jackets

Belted tunics

Skirts with wide waistbands

If you have a long torso or waist:

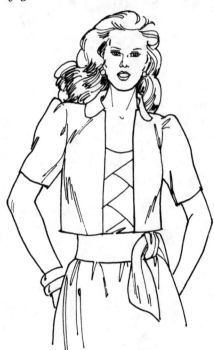

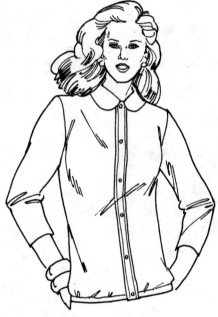

Yes to:

Unfitted or empire styles

High-rise slacks (straight leg falling over shoe)

Wide belts; cummerbunds

Separates

Short-waisted jackets

High-heeled shoes

No to:

Low-rise pants

Dropped waistlines

Belts worn low on waist

Overblouses and blousons

Long-waisted jackets

Hip huggers

Tops with strong vertical designs

Short hemlines

Narrow belts

*If you have
a small bust:*

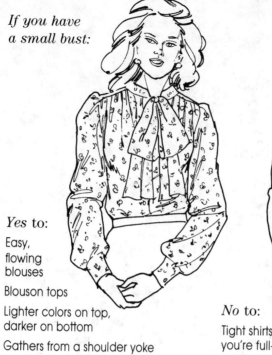

Yes to:

Easy,
flowing
blouses

Blouson tops

Lighter colors on top,
darker on bottom

Gathers from a shoulder yoke

Front interest: large, soft bow or jabot

Patch pockets

A good support bra

Longer, slightly flared A-line or
straight skirts

No to:

Tight shirts, especially if
you're full-hipped

Clingy tops

V-necks

Ribbed sweaters

If you have a thick waist:

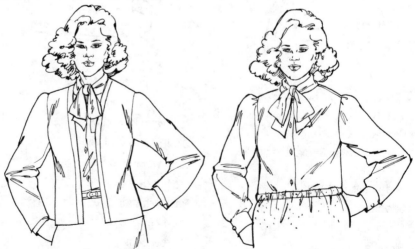

Yes to:

Chanel-type jackets

Blouson waists that drop somewhat

Vests

Loose waistlines

Belts worn on hips

Tunic tops

Slacks with pleats

Unfitted jackets

Blouson-style shirts, dresses

Focusing attention away from waist

Chemises, long lines

Wide or wrap belts (test them!)

Princess styles

No to:

Nipped-in waists

Skirts that pleat or gather at waist

Tucked-in blouses

Thick, clingy fabrics

If you have a small waist: **Make the most (or least) of it!**

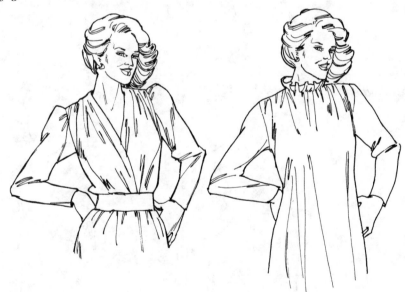

Yes to:

Nipped-in waists

Belted tunics

Belts which focus attention on waist

No to:

Exaggerated blouson styles

Unbelted tunics

Shapeless dresses

Vests which cover sides of waist

If you have a swayback:

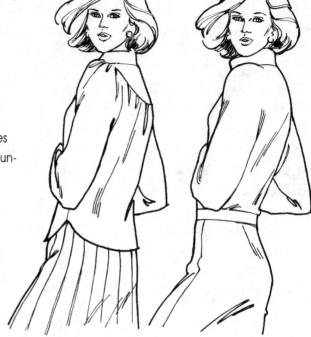

Yes to:

Overblouses, jackets with unfitted waistlines

Skirts with gathers or un-pressed pleats

No to:

Tight skirts or pants

If your abdomen protrudes:

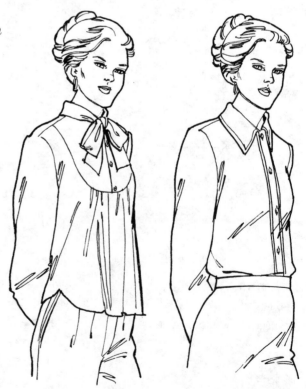

Yes to:

Overblouses which hang softly over abdomen

A-line skirts

Trousers with soft pleats

Chemises and other loose-fitting, waistless dresses

Side-slash pockets

Skirts with stitched-down pleats over stomach (for a girdle effect)

Seven-gore skirts

No to:

Straight or gored skirts

Clingy fabrics, knits

Tight belts

Tight pants

Gathered, full skirts

If you have a flat derriere:

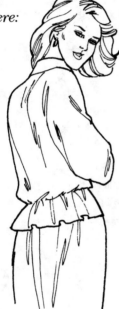 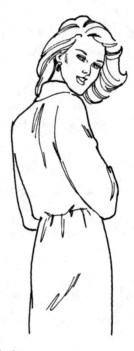

Yes to:

Two-piece dresses

Gathered skirts

Hip pockets

Seams in pants which run from back darts down center back of leg (eliminates bagginess)

Short vests

No to:

One-piece knits

Tight, form-fitting dresses or skirts

Straight skirts

If you have a large derriere:

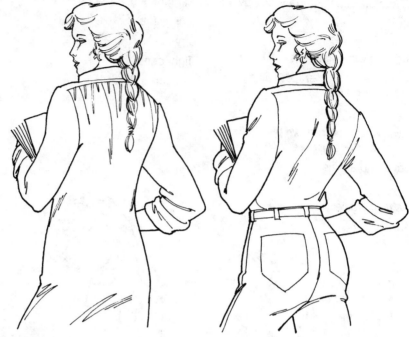

Yes to:

Garments which fall from the shoulders or arms in uninterrupted lines: caftans, chemises

Long vests

Dirndls and softly pleated skirts

No to:

Too-tight pants

Clingy pants or skirts

Tuck-in shirts

Figure-hugging knits

If your hips are heavy:

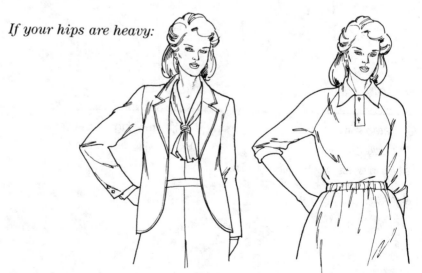

Yes to:

Inverted-pleat A-line skirt

Focus attention on upper body with scarves, color, jewelry

Sewn-down wide-pleated skirt (gives abdomen control, too)

Broader shoulder lines

Cardigan jacket

Unbuttoned jacket with pants

Straight wrap skirt (focuses a vertical line which is only 3/4 width of hip)

Button-front A-line skirts

Loose-fitting slacks

Seamless pants

Chanel jacket

Pea jacket

Gored skirt

Dark skirts, pants; lighter tops

Duller finish fabrics

Skirts that hug top of hips and fall gently

Skirts and slacks in simple designs

No to:

Large plaids

Broad horizontal stripes

Narrow shoulder lines

Clingy, fitted tops

Wide belts or any waistline interest, even if waist is small

Dirndl skirts

Below-waistline trim or detail

Straight, front-slit skirts

Straight pleated skirts

Kilts

Wide-wale corduroy

Tight slacks

Lightweight fabrics that cling

Over-the-knee boots

Loud-colored bottoms

Back pockets

Front pleated pants

Fitted peplum jacket

Patch pockets on pants or skirts

If your hips are too narrow:

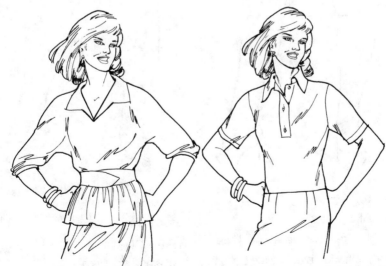

Yes to:

Belted overblouses

Peg-topped skirts

Pants with pleats

Gathered waistlines

Substantial weight fabrics

Pants with side pockets

No to:

Blouson tops

Form-fitting garments

Tightly fitted pants, skirts

Hip huggers

If you're wondering about hem lengths:

Yes, generally, to:

Skirts ending about an inch below the knee (unless you're very tall and long-legged; you could then go to mid-calf).

Note: If you wear very high heels or a draping dress, you can use a longer skirt.

Heavier, lower heels balance best with a shorter skirt.

No to:

Skirts which end at the widest part of the leg. (Wear them just below the widest point, unless you are very short or have very thin legs.)

If your legs are heavy:

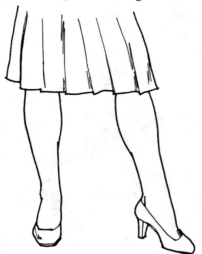
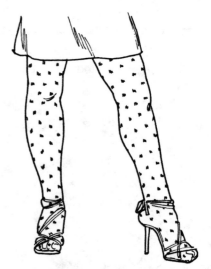

Yes to:

Straight-leg slacks

Straight dirndl skirts, worn over knee

Shorts with wide pleats, wide bottoms

No to:

Short skirts

Extra-tight pants

Patterned stockings

Clothes which keep eye focused above waist

Light-colored tops (draw eye to face)

Semifitted jackets

Culotte skirts (substitute for pants)

Simple shoes with low vamp

Boots

Matching shoes, hose, skirt

Simple espadrilles with wedge

Closed-toe pumps

Two- to three-inch heels, but not too narrow

White or very light stockings

Dainty shoes, sandals

Spike heels

If you have skinny legs:

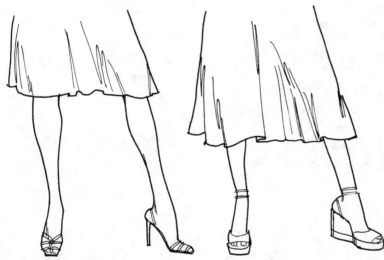

Yes to:

Knee-length hems

Light-colored hose

Skirts which end at the widest part of your leg

Low-heel barefoot sandals

Small-scale, light-weight shoes

Dainty, simple pumps

Light, strappy sandals

Thin high heels

No to:

Skirts too long or too short

Dark hose

Socks with bulky cuffs

Clunky shoes

If your legs are very short:

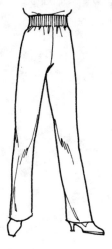
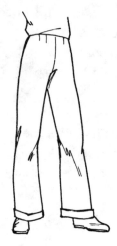

Yes to:

Vertical lines

Loose trousers (long, straight leg which falls over shoe)

Waist above natural waistline

One color, head to toe (accents OK, for interest)

Higher heeled shoes

Long skirts with boots

Bathing suits cut high on hips

No to:

Hip-hugger pants

Peg-leg pants

Low-riding belts

Wide prints or plaids

Horizontal stripes

Bulky, textured pants or skirts which add dimension

Thick, wide-wale corduroy

Dropped waist

Full skirt

I know this is an overwhelming amount of material to absorb. But I hope you will refer to it again and again, because these ideas for cooperating *with* the shape God gave you, rather than fighting against it, really do work.

When Sharon, one of our consultants, analyzed her figure, she realized that although she had thought she had large hips, she actually had heavy legs and narrow shoulders. She was a classic T-shape. At a recent seminar, she looked wonderful in a dress with puffed sleeves to widen her shoulders and balance her thighs, and dark stockings to minimize her lower legs. Her proportions *looked* perfect.

Many women are asked if they've lost weight after they begin using slenderizing illusions in their dress.

Carol, a client who wanted to emphasize her tiny waist, began to realize that in doing so, she called attention to her large hips. She, too, learned to broaden her shoulders and finally realized that she should de-emphasize her waist to make her hips appear slimmer.

A woman with a dowager's hump who was wearing clingy fabrics seemed to be saying to the world, "Here's my back and this is what it looks like." She was so pleased when I showed her the difference it made to wear a collar which stood away from the back of her neck.

The women who seem to have the greatest problem are the large breasted. They're inevitably delighted when I show them a vertical neckline and soft front treatment which gives them room to hide under.

And what about my "bird head"? Why, I keep my hair full to widen my head, so that it balances with my long body. (And you'd better believe that I cover those knees that smile at each other!)

It's often said that beauty is in the eye of the beholder. I hope you're beginning to see that's precisely what happens when you show pleasing lines to the beholder's eye. He or she can see you as thinner or rounder, taller or shorter than you really are.

It's not "faking it," but simply revealing the best of yourself and using the lines of your clothing to enhance the wonderful body which is special and unique.

BEAUTY IS STYLE

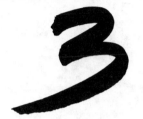

BEING UNIQUELY YOU

Your spiritual style. In his office, the plastic surgeon proudly displayed "before" and "after" pictures of rhinoplasty patients. They would come to him with noses of astonishing variety—some grotesque, some just large enough to have "character." The surgeon's skill had left all of them with a rubber-stamp sameness; all had darling little catlike nose profiles.

Of course, as adolescents, we wanted to be like everyone else. But aren't you glad now, that God hasn't stamped us out in such monotonous uniformity, either physically or spiritually?

It's so special for me to know that there is no one in all the world just like me. Just as no two snowflakes are alike, both you and I are "originals," endowed with our own particular spiritual sensitivities and sensibilities, our own temperament and talents.

And we can rest in the knowledge that he knew precisely what he was doing. "Thy hands fashioned and made me," Job affirms. And in Psalm 139, David expresses how God formed our inward parts, knit each of us in our mother's womb. In Psalm 8:5, he declares that God made us a little lower than the angels; and in 17:8, he implores God to keep him as "the apple of [his] eye."

We are the apple of his eye, of great worth to him. And it seems to me that our worth lies, at least in part, in our uniqueness.

Look at the assortment of biblical men and women God created and used to his glory: from the reluctant Moses to the overachiever Saul; from the gentle, self-effacing Mary, mother of Jesus, to the energetic Priscilla. Consider the unlikely mix of characters Jesus gathered as his apostles, from foot-in-the-mouth Peter to show-me Thomas.

It's exciting to begin to understand and appreciate the unique persons we are.

Now it's true that we may not be "gifted" in the sense of the school child who is identified as such on the basis of specific tests. But each of us is endowed with certain talents, certain natural learning. Often, it's not at all a matter of education or training, but rather, an attitude of the heart.

Have you considered what your gifts might be? Here's a check list which might help you to discover some you've not thought of before.

_____ I truly enjoy doing things for other people, whether it's serving them coffee or dinner at my home, or assisting when they're in a time-bind.

_____ I'm the one who frequently volunteers to drive someone to a meeting, or take dinner to someone who is ill.

_____ I appear to have a knack for showing others how to do specific tasks or to learn certain arts.

_____ I like to analyze things and I find I can simplify and clarify complicated ideas and concepts for other people.

_____ I'm often able to see problem areas which others may overlook.

_____ I love to encourage and motivate others to do worthwhile things.

_____ I'm an idea person with a good bit of imagination. I love to pioneer new projects.

_____ When I see a financial need, I'm one of the first to give as much as I can.

_____ I seem to be able to earn and manage money well, and I'm grateful for opportunities to share it.

_____ I'm good with my hands and find great satisfaction in making things.

_____ I'm an effective organizer and I love to make things run smoothly.

_____ Though I'm not in an executive position, people ask my advice whenever there's a project to be planned.

_____ I'm not an innovator, but I love to coordinate and keep existing structures functioning well.

I'm sure you've checked some of these points—probably several. So, you see, you _are_ gifted!

The Bible identifies our special spiritual gifts as serving, teaching, exhorting or encouraging, giving money, assisting others, and administration. And it makes it clear that the magnitude of the gift is not important. (1 Corinthians 12:22 tells us that, "Those parts of the body that seem to be weaker are indispensable.")

We'll recognize these gifts because they allow us to function not with gritted-teeth, guess-I'd-better-do-it determination, but with an uncontrived and natural ease which flows from our innermost beings.

Then we will know the sense of rightness which comes from being who we really are. Like Esther, who blossomed and served most profoundly and compellingly when she followed Mordecai's counsel to be herself and reveal herself, we too, will function most effectively.

Some of us will speak eloquently to large groups, while others are most effective on a one-to-one basis. Some can open our homes to any number of people on short notice. Others will find that the elderly widow on our block loves our homemade soup. Perhaps we'll have a talent for organizing an entire corporation, or for leading a junior high group's ski trip. Some of us will excel as encouragers to others and others will be gifted at making money—and sharing it well.

The Lord can effectively use a variety of people. (The body is able to move and walk and talk and reach out when it is made up of all the proper parts, not when it is all arms and legs—or mouths.)

What part of the body do you sense that you are? If you're not sure, consider what opportunities seem to come to you again and again.

I would urge you to decide now to be a specialist. But, you say, developing many skills is good! True, but we can stretch in only one direction, or we will become very much out of shape.

I find I do much better when I don't try to be like everyone else, when I concentrate on what *I* do best. It's so much more satisfying and effective than the scatter-shot approach of doing a lot of things half-well.

My challenge to you, then, is to dare to focus and to excel. (Suggested reading: Romans 12:6-8; 1 Corinthians 12.)

Your outer style. Just as we each have certain innate gifts which give us our own unique inner "style," we each have our own natural external style preferences. I call it our personality style type.

Part of it is our nature—the way we were created. And part of it stems from nurture—how we were raised, how others see us.

It begins in our earliest years. I was a delicate blonde child, and my mother dressed me in ruffles. Boys strove to protect me and I was to hear, "Now, don't bother your pretty head over that," many times. I loved modeling for TV as a child and always wanted to look perfect.

My co-author, Bev, on the other hand, was a wiry, brown-haired child who complained the very day she received her first roller skates that they weren't fast enough. Her mother didn't dare dress her in ruffles. They might get in the way of Bev's tree-climbing!

We are also profoundly influenced by others' expectations of us. Have you ever heard of the Pygmalion effect? It's a fascinating psychological concept which states that if I expect certain things of you, you very often will act to fulfill my expectations. A simple example: If I tell my child she'll never amount to anything, chances are very great that she will not.

In one study, male students telephoned female students. Some of the females had been labeled beforehand as attractive, some as not. The women did not know how they'd been defined. Still, those who were said to be attractive seemed to the men to be witty and interesting over the phone. The others sounded dull.

They had fulfilled the men's expectations.

We tend to do this in selecting the styles we wear. We respond to old expectations of our mothers, or perhaps to more current projections from others.

Sometimes they are contrary to our nature, and we feel uneasy, but don't understand why.

Each of us has a basic personality style type. It's an essence or air or feeling about us. It's more than just a matter of preference, but a whole countenance. If you're tuned in to your own style, it's evident in your taste, your likes and dislikes. If you dress to express your personality, you feel comfortable, and others feel at ease around you. If you don't, even though you look "put together" in your dress, you may not be believable to others. It's subtle; most people will not understand why they feel confusion or lack of trust when a woman's style of dressing doesn't reflect who she really is.

Think a moment about different style types in the entertainment world. Picture, for instance, Cher, with all her flamboyance. Now picture the simple, youthful-looking Sandra Dee.

Now imagine Cher in a preppy plaid skirt and a shirt with a Peter Pan collar and a tiny bow at the neck. Imagine Sandra Dee in a slinky, form-fitting sequin-covered gown with a jacket made of feathers. It just doesn't fit, does it?

As women begin to recognize these basic style differences as they attend my Uniquely You classes, I inevitably hear a great

"Aha!" of recognition and relief. For instance, I remember a young woman in an expensive tailored suit. Many of the other women there would have loved to own it. But she hated it. "My husband always shops with me when I go to buy clothes," she explained. "He's a banker. Can't you tell?"

"I would love to look terribly elegant," admitted another woman. "When I was eleven years old and five feet eight inches tall, my mother told me again and again, 'Tall people can look so elegant!' The problem is, I'm a casual person. I have trouble keeping my shoes on."

"I'm not sure *what* I like," confessed a teenager who wore a frilly blouse with her jeans. "And styles change so quickly. What I bought last year looks silly this season."

I've found through the years that women fall into six basic style types. Yet because they don't realize this, they are pulled by the dictates of fashion or by the opinions of other people and many never really achieve their own identity.

This chapter is not an attempt to box you in, or pigeonhole you, but is designed to help you find your own personality style type, based upon your own preferences. Then you will be able to choose clothes which make you feel most comfortable.

Choosing your preferences from the following lists will help you discover what garments express you most accurately, how to be true to yourself and to be the very best you are—not something you aren't. Probably you will find that you check several different categories, but that you are strongest in one, or possibly two.

Remember, too, your style type is not cast in cement. It will possibly change as you mature.

PERSONAL STYLE QUESTIONNAIRE

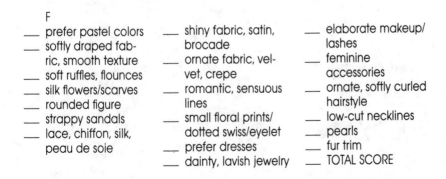

F
___ prefer pastel colors
___ softly draped fabric, smooth texture
___ soft ruffles, flounces
___ silk flowers/scarves
___ rounded figure
___ strappy sandals
___ lace, chiffon, silk, peau de soie

___ shiny fabric, satin, brocade
___ ornate fabric, velvet, crepe
___ romantic, sensuous lines
___ small floral prints/ dotted swiss/eyelet
___ prefer dresses
___ dainty, lavish jewelry

___ elaborate makeup/ lashes
___ feminine accessories
___ ornate, softly curled hairstyle
___ low-cut necklines
___ pearls
___ fur trim
___ TOTAL SCORE

C

- ___ average balanced figure
- ___ classic refined look
- ___ soft, straight lines/fullness
- ___ w/pleats or folds
- ___ tailored lines/conservative
- ___ matte-finish, smooth fabric
- ___ light-weight fabric
- ___ fine cotton, crepe, silk
- ___ medium prints, stripes
- ___ costume ensembles
- ___ prefer skirted suits
- ___ soft, controlled hair
- ___ moderate makeup
- ___ simple elegant jewelry
- ___ classic shoes, pumps
- ___ tweed, wool
- ___ moderate, muted prints, or solids
- ___ complete coordinated look
- ___ pin stripe/club print
- ___ TOTAL SCORE

Y

- ___ small stature
- ___ gentle, rounded figure
- ___ dainty, delicate look
- ___ prefer neutral colors
- ___ soft curved lines
- ___ bows/ribbons
- ___ hand-woven prints
- ___ cashmere, angora
- ___ crisp cotton, voile
- ___ eyelet, thin jersey
- ___ youthful, unsophisticated styling
- ___ dainty, simple jewelry
- ___ soft woolens
- ___ Victorian style
- ___ curvy hairstyle/wedge cut
- ___ minimal makeup
- ___ two piece dresses
- ___ TOTAL SCORE

D

- ___ angular features
- ___ severe straight lines
- ___ billowy, blousy
- ___ bouffant, crisp lines
- ___ piping, buttons, contrast trim
- ___ crisp stand-up ruffles
- ___ fur trim
- ___ shiny, glittery fabrics
- ___ exotic colors/prints
- ___ lavishly ornate fabrics
- ___ large prints, geometrics
- ___ bold, large, abstract, modern jewelry
- ___ elaborate makeup
- ___ severe, plain hairstyle
- ___ tight, curly perm
- ___ long, bright nails
- ___ ethnic look (stylish design)
- ___ satin, heavy brocade, velvet
- ___ velour, nylon, jersey
- ___ theatrical look
- ___ prefer contrasting colors
- ___ TOTAL SCORE

T

- ___ average to tall, broad features
- ___ sturdy athletic figure
- ___ elegant sportswear
- ___ denim, khaki
- ___ prefer separates
- ___ outdoor casual, sporty look
- ___ casual, sporty look
- ___ plaids, checks, paisleys
- ___ broad features
- ___ rough, nubby, matte-finish fabric
- ___ crepe, raw silk, quilting
- ___ penny loafers
- ___ corduroy, tweeds, all-over prints
- ___ large, casual design
- ___ rough linen, crisp cotton
- ___ simple, handmade jewelry
- ___ large chains
- ___ minimal makeup, "natural look"
- ___ casual/wash & walk hairstyle
- ___ boots, casual walking shoes
- ___ prefer earth tones
- ___ gabardine, plain knits
- ___ TOTAL SCORE

P

- understated elegance
- sturdy, not fragile figure
- skirt and sweater sets
- checks, plaids, stripes
- preppy style
- casual, natural look
- gingham, piqué
- ribbon ties

- linen, tweeds
- corduroy
- walking shorts
- crest buttons
- jersey, knits
- vest sets
- Peter Pan collars
- emblems, monograms
- minimal jewelry

- T-shirt tops
- simple chains, pins, rings
- natural, windblown hairstyle
- sportswear
- prefer separates
- TOTAL SCORE

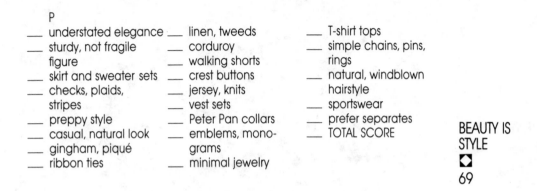
If you score highest in the "F" category, you are primarily a *Feminine/Romantic.* You might be like Jaclyn Smith—soft, feminine, with a delicate essence. Or you might be more like Zsa Zsa Gabor—more theatrically romantic, with a sensuous flair. You spend time on your makeup, nails. You may not own a pair of jeans! Ruth, a very feminine woman of the Bible, was probably a Feminine/Romantic.

If you have more check marks in the "C" classification, you are a *Classic/Sophisticate,* a "city" person, as contrasted with the "country" look. Barbara Walters is an example of the no-nonsense, somewhat reserved approach of the cool, collected sophisticate. Nancy Reagan is the classic counterpart—timeless, conservative, tailored.

In the Bible, Miriam, a born leader, and Lydia, a very independent woman, could have been Classic/Sophisticates.

"Y" is for *Youthful Romantic.* You have always looked younger than you actually are, and probably always will. The look is understated, unsophisticated. You're sparkly—perhaps a bit naive. Debbie Reynolds and Goldie Hawn are Youthful/Romantics.

"D" is for *Dramatic,* and you may very well be an amateur or professional entertainer, or work in some facet of the beauty business. Some of you are avant garde, love the exotic and extreme—like Cher Bono. Others are poised, self-assured, but quiet and reserved—like Marlene Dietrich. In biblical times, Bathsheba may have been a Dramatic; and possibly Rachel, since Jacob was so captivated by her beauty the moment he saw her.

"T" is for *Town and Country/Natural.* The Town and Country is the most sophisticated emphasis of this style type—rather elegant,

(continued on p. 76)

FEMININE/ROMANTIC

prefers pastel colors

softly draped fabric, smooth texture

soft ruffles, flounces

silk flowers/scarves

rounded figure

strappy sandals

lace, chiffon, silk, peau de soie

shiny fabric, satin, brocade

ornate fabric, velvet, crepe

romantic, sensuous lines

small floral prints/dotted swiss/eyelet

prefers dresses

dainty, lavish jewelry

elaborate makeup/lashes

feminine accessories

ornate, softly curled hairstyle

low-cut necklines

pearls

fur trim

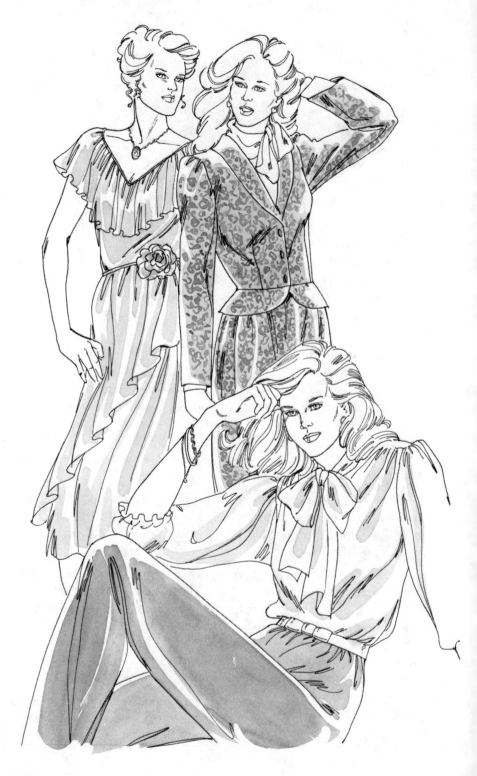

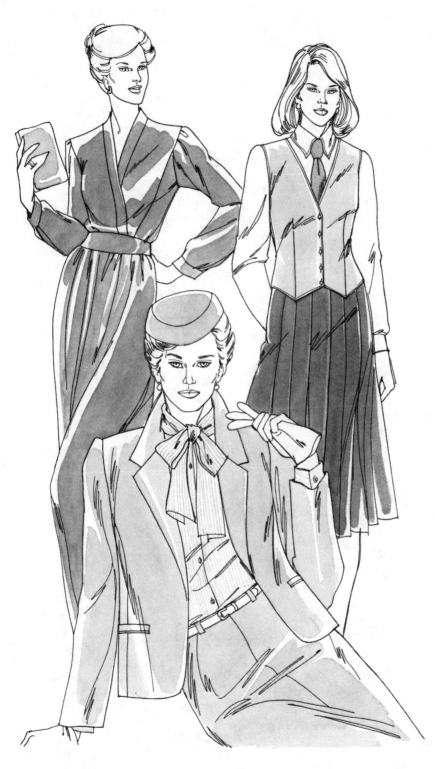

CLASSIC/
SOPHISTICATE

average balanced
figure

classic refined look

soft straight lines/fullness
w/pleats or folds

tailored lines/conserva-
tive

matte-finish, smooth
fabric

light-weight fabric

fine cotton, crepe, silk

medium prints, stripes

costume ensembles

prefers skirted suits

soft, controlled hair

moderate makeup

simple, elegant jewelry

classic shoes, pumps

tweed, wool

moderate, muted prints
or solids

complete coordinated
look

pin stripe/club print

YOUTHFUL ROMANTIC

small stature

gentle, rounded figure

dainty, delicate look

prefers neutral colors

soft curved lines

bows/ribbons

hand-woven prints

cashmere, angora

crisp cotton, voile

eyelet, thin jersey

youthful, unsophisti-
cated styling

dainty, simple jewelry

soft woolens

Victorian style

curvy, hairstyle/wedge
cut

minimal makeup

two piece dresses

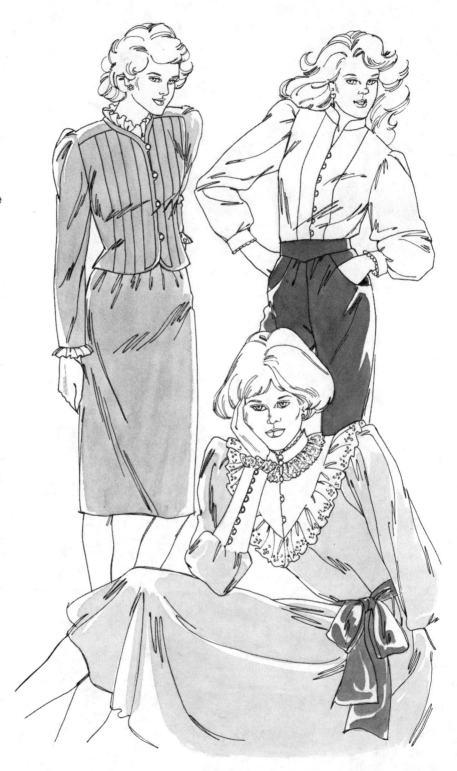

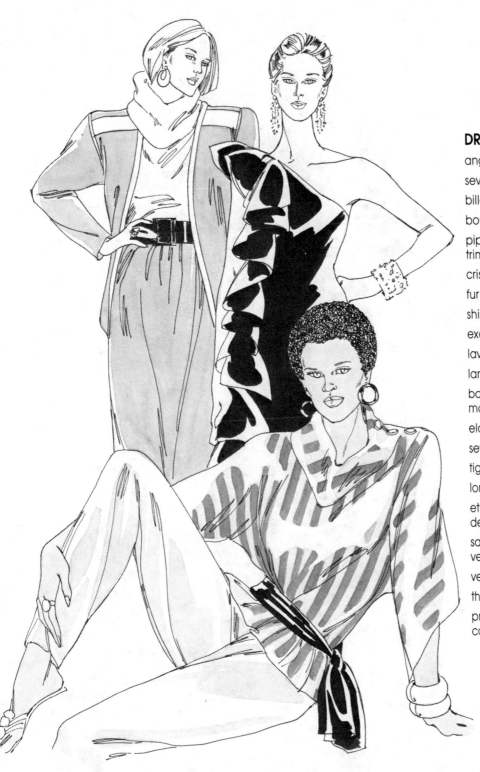

DRAMATIC

angular features

severe straight lines

billowy, blousy

bouffant, crisp lines

piping, buttons, contrast trim

crisp stand-up ruffles

fur trim

shiny, glittery fabrics

exotic colors/prints

lavishly ornate fabrics

large prints, geometrics

bold, large, abstract, modern jewelry

elaborate makeup

severe, plain hairstyle

tight, curly perm

long, bright nails

ethnic look (stylish design)

satin, heavy brocade, velvet

velour, nylon, jersey

theatrical look

prefers contrasting colors

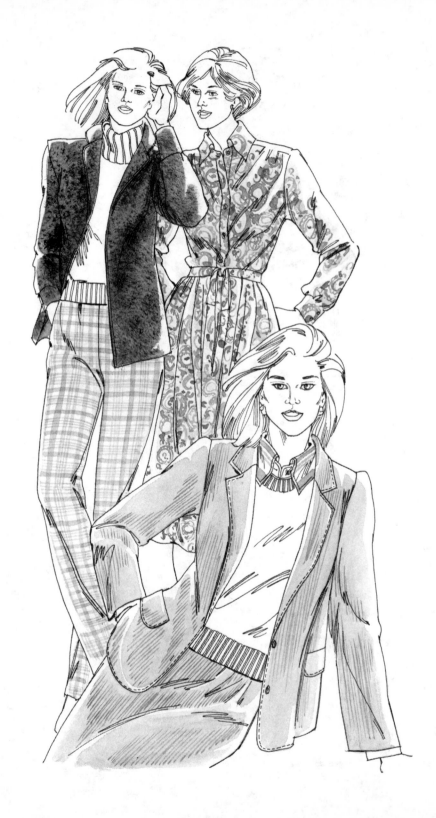

TOWN AND COUNTRY/NATURAL

average to tall

sturdy athletic figure

elegant sportswear

denim, khaki

prefers separates

outdoor casual, sporty look

casual, sporty look

plaids, checks, paisleys

broad features

rough, nubby, matte-finish fabric

crepe, raw silk, quilting

penny loafers

corduroy, tweeds, all-over prints

large, casual design

rough linen, crisp cotton

simple, handmade jewelry

large chains

minimal makeup, "natural look"

casual/wash & walk hairstyle

boots, casual walking shoe

prefers earth tones

gabardine, plain knits

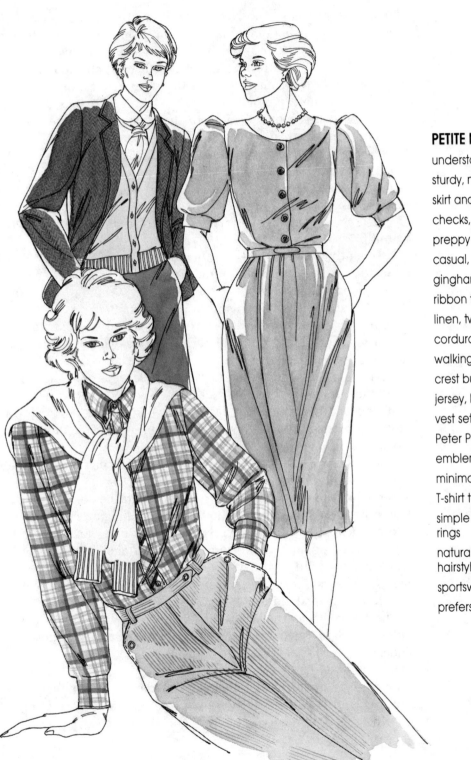

PETITE NATURAL

- understated elegance
- sturdy, not fragile figure
- skirt and sweater sets
- checks, plaids, stripes
- preppy style
- casual, natural look
- gingham, piqué
- ribbon ties
- linen, tweeds
- corduroy
- walking shorts
- crest buttons
- jersey, knits
- vest sets
- Peter Pan collar
- emblems, monograms
- minimal jewelry
- T-shirt tops
- simple chains, pins, rings
- natural, windblown hairstyle
- sportswear
- prefers separates

like Jackie Kennedy. The Natural tends to be casual and prefers pants, sportswear, minimal makeup. Carol Burnett is a contemporary example. Rebekah in the Bible may have been this type—the "doer" who was very beautiful, yet healthy and strong enough to draw water for ten camels. (That's thirty to sixty gallons of water, according to one camel authority!)

Perhaps you responded most to the P group. You are a *Petite Natural*, which is really a mini Town and Country/Natural. You may be slender, but not fragile; sturdy, but not large in build. You are young at heart, perky, alert, effervescent, and natural. Your manner is casual with perhaps a touch of the tomboy. You like a natural look, dislike fussing with your hair, and are very likely tanned or freckled. Sandy Duncan and Sally Field are examples of the Petite Natural.

Frequently we'll see these combinations: Feminine/Romantic and Dramatic; Youthful Romantic and Feminine/Romantic; Feminine/ Romantic and Classic/Sophisticate; Town and Country/Natural and Petite Natural; Classic/Sophisticate and Dramatic.

If you've checked your style preferences and still are not sure "what you are," try clipping pictures of styles you like from magazines and newspapers for a month. Or get an outdated pattern book from a fabric store and mark the styles you enjoy. You'll see that your preferences tend to fall into one or two categories.

If you test high in many categories, take a long look at your clothes. Try them on, one by one. Stand in front of the mirror and ask yourself, "How does this feel? Is this really me?"

I once knew a young woman who thought she could be anything she wanted to be, and dressed accordingly. One day she'd wear a severely tailored, oxford gray three-piece suit; the next, a full, harlequin patterned skirt and a blouse with a plunging neckline. She adopted a totally different hairstyle every week. Now, you might think she was simply exercising freedom of choice, following the way she felt on different days. But ultimately, it didn't ring true with her co-workers. As one man expressed it, "Who *is* Julia? Will the real Julia please stand up?"

The tragedy was that *she* didn't know who the real Julia was, either. She later spent years in therapy after having attempted suicide.

So, much as many of us resist being "typed," there really is a style or style-combination which is most appropriate and most natural for you. If you're still not sure, try out some different styles on others. Notice the reactions you get.

One of my consultants, Cam, dressed in a Town and Country mode for years, but tested high in a classic-conservative category. When she wore a more sophisticated style to her husband's company Christmas party, many failed to recognize her. She found people gathering around her all evening. The feedback was clear; she felt her "new look" made her more credible, more believable as a person.

However, as helpful as others' reactions may be, you must learn to trust yourself. Trust your intuition. You'll find you know more than you think you do. Then you'll have the freedom to zero in on who *you* really are—not the person your friend is, not the person the stores or ads or fashion shows tell you you should be, not the person your mother or husband or sister says you should be.

As you think about your clothes, you may find that you are in process, evolving from one style type to another. Most girls are Youthful Romantics, or possibly Petite Naturals. And many women who were Feminine/Romantics in their teens and twenties may gradually move toward the Classic/Sophisticate. Thus your clothing history may very well be your own personal history, as you grow and mature.

Uniquely You has seen dramatic changes in women's lives when they begin to perceive themselves accurately, confirming that our clothing affects how people perceive us.

Eileen, single for eighteen adulthood years, had no men at all in her life. When she came to Uniquely You, her clothing was a mixture of many style types. Then she recognized herself as a Romantic and began to dress in soft fabrics, to allow herself the feminine details in clothing that she really loved. As she felt more herself, more free, she stopped hiding. And soon, she found a number of men attracted to her.

(If you're single, as you discover your style type, notice which men you attract. We'll tell you more about this in chapter 5.)

Marj, a new USC graduate, was accustomed to conforming to the sportive style of her friends in college. Denims, plaids, T-shirts, and little makeup were her hallmarks. But she found it difficult to land the job for which she trained until she "packaged" herself as the Classic/Sophisticate style type, which was the "real" Marj. The difference? Now she more closely conformed to the "successful career" look of the company she wished to join.

And by the way, many offices still have their own "uniform," although I'm glad to see that this is changing. However, if you work for such a corporation and wish to move ahead, be sure you understand that uniform. You can be true to your style type, but you may have to tone it down a bit to look believable to others in your job—or in the job to which you'd like to be promoted. (We'll tell you more about this in chapter 8.)

Now, while "conforming" was comfortable for Marj, this is not always the case. For instance, a home economist who was a Petite Natural came to me seeking a makeover because she thought she wanted to change careers and go into a bank executive training program.

Of course, I'm not a career counselor. But it struck me that both her style type and her current job were probably exactly right for her. I suggested that she think it over carefully before making the change, and she ultimately decided to stay with what she knew and, in her heart, really loved.

DRESSING FOR THE MAN IN YOUR LIFE

At the end of almost every lecture I give on personality style types, someone asks, "What if my husband likes me in ruffles and I hate them?" Or, someone has a dilemma similar to the woman we mentioned earlier, whose husband dressed her like a banker.

I urge women to share these differences honestly with their husbands, to show them that, just as there are different personalities in this world, there are different basic style types.

Often, they've worked out compromises. For instance, when natural-looking Karen was told by her husband that he wanted her to look more romantic, he wasn't really looking for lace and frills. He simply wanted her to wear skirts more often and to be a little more caring about her appearance.

On the other hand, romantic Gail's husband thought she always looked too dressed up and wondered why she couldn't wear jeans occasionally. She was able to explain to him how uncomfortable she felt in stiff denim pants, and he agreed to settle for casual wrap skirts and culottes.

Another question women frequently ask me is whether it's possible to remain true to your own style no matter what type of activity you're involved in. Definitely. And it's important. Because if you don't dress compatibly with your style type, you'll feel uncomfortable. On the other hand, if you don't consider the circumstances, you may make others feel uncomfortable. It's thoughtful and courteous to adjust.

A woman in a seminar once told of her dilemma. She was a

Classic/Sophisticate, but her husband manufactured fishing equipment and she frequently went fly-fishing with him. I showed her how to find neatly tailored, color-coordinated pants, hat, and top, which are totally in keeping with her classic image, but also appropriate for the activity.

Even the Feminine/Romantic can be herself at a casual affair without looking overdressed, as Gail discovered. And she'll also find plenty of feminine touches when she looks for active sportwear: lacy trims on tennis togs, eyelet-edged sun-visors, ruffles on swimsuits.

Moreover, the Town and Country/Natural can look absolutely smashing at a formal affair. She uses simple lines and elegantly textured fabrics which are true to her nature but totally in keeping with the occasion.

God created each of us *individually*, without the use of cookie cutters, photocopiers, or cloning. Take the time to discover the styles which are uniquely, comfortably your own. You'll feel better, look better, and be more confident. And you'll be believable because you are expressing yourself honestly. Make the effort to be the very best that *you* are!

BEAUTY IS HARMONY

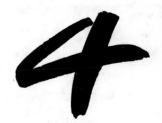

CHAPTER 4

YIELDING TO THE HARMONY OF GOD'S PLAN FOR US

While I was in college, I traveled with "The Sonlight" singing group, and I never failed to marvel at how well our performances came together. When we warmed up, in rehearsal, we really sounded dreadful; often we were jarringly out of tune. But after we had vocalized for awhile, what a difference! Every note came together in a satisfying, connected wholeness.

That is the harmony, magnified to infinity, which we find when we bring the "notes" of our lives into harmony.

And this is the harmony I feel about what I'm doing today. People ask me how I can carry on such a full and sometimes "hectic" schedule without coming unhinged. Well, it's because I know I'm doing exactly what I was designed to do, and because I have never forced it, but have let the work grow naturally.

I think I particularly appreciate this harmony today, because I have known what it is for my life to be "off key." In fact, a number of years ago, I reacted to this tension by becoming agoraphobic. As a typical victim of this disorder, which means literally, "fear of the marketplace," I had such fears of going out that I couldn't leave the house. I was paralyzed by the fear of fear, the fear of panicking, the fear of leaving my "comfort zone."

And yet I know now that even though I felt a million miles away from the Lord at that time, he didn't leave me for a moment. Everything was in the plan—because Uniquely You would never have started if I hadn't suffered from agoraphobia. During the time I was totally housebound, there was little to do but read. And I devoured everything I could find on color, line, image, clothes, makeup.

Gradually, through counseling, I became aware that I was running and hiding because I was afraid of my own power. Then, finally, I was able to redirect all this energy and combine all my research with my past experience to found Uniquely You. (This experience included modeling—a public relations job in which I traveled around the country for several companies; and working as a Revlon makeup artist.)

My new corporation began to catch on almost immediately. Soon, four different people approached me to write a business plan, urging me to expand the company. And, at the same time, my parents cautioned me to stay small. They were afraid expansion would create so much pressure, I'd surely die at a very tender age.

As I struggled with the decision, I realized that what was right was to leave it strictly to the Lord to direct us. I said, "Lord, I'm not going to do anything to promote this, but whatever opportunities you lay in front of me, I will follow through on."

More and more people came to me, with larger and larger accounts. And more and more women called, seeking training as consultants.

I knew if I forced the company's growth, it would be unnatural and overwhelming. So as the work seemed to gently progress, I just flowed with it. I was alert, it's true, to what needed to be done. I was always responding to opportunities and needs, but watching in wonderment as it all unfolded.

So many of us search and search for harmony in our lives. We yearn for it. Yet we just can't seem to do it on our own, no matter how carefully we plan. Sometimes, in a desperate attempt to bring it all together, we flock to self-improvement, human potential seminars, telling ourselves, "I'm OK. Here I'll find the answers to taking charge of my life."

But each hopeful, this-will-do-it attempt seems eventually to drop us either into unrest or confusion and despair.

If we truly surrender to God and ask his guidance, we find such sweet harmony in "letting go and letting God." We begin to realize that not only is he totally able; he is *the* adequate resource for our lives.

God knows us better than we know ourselves. He has wisdom and insight into the big picture of what's best for us.

Yielding doesn't mean twiddling our thumbs and waiting for "revelation," or to be turned on like robots. We seek the sovereign direction of the Bible. We use our common sense and wait for that divine inner feedback which either gives us a sense of confirmation and peace, or an inner "uh-uh" sense of denial.

It does mean trusting him to help us achieve an overall balance in our lives and to show us when it's time to back off on one area and concentrate on another.

And that means trusting him even though sometimes his plan doesn't seem logical to us. Do you, for instance, suppose that Joshua's army thought God's plan for the taking of Jericho was logical? I mean, really—marching around the city for seven days and blowing trumpets! But it worked.

Certainly my agoraphobia didn't make sense to me at the time. But now, with 20/20 hindsight, I can thank God for that pain, and, in fact, for everything I've ever gone through. Now I see that it has all been part of his plan for my growth.

I am so grateful for the sense of peace and harmony I have about what I am doing today, and it's a great joy to me when I see others also discover it.

Many of my consultants tell me they had been searching for the right occupation and that they truly felt led to us.

He will show you the path of your life, too, if you will trust him.

Perhaps you'd like to read some Scripture verses which describe how masterfully he does this.

One of my favorites is Psalm 16:11.

You have made known to me the path of life;
you will fill me with joy in your presence,
with eternal pleasures at your right hand.

Turn, too, to Proverbs 3:6, Matthew 3:3, Hebrews 12:13, and John 14:6.

LEARNING THE HARMONY OF GOD'S COLOR PLAN FOR YOU

One way to bring harmony to our outward appearance—and certainly the most visible way—is through the use of color.

Surely, God loves color. He endowed the birds with a rainbow of colors, from the iridescent greens and reds of the hummingbird to the brilliant blues of the jays; from the russet of a robin's breast to the striking yellow of the canary. And so colorfully did he create our fruits and flowers, we've appropriated their names to describe colors: grape, peach, apricot, orange, pumpkin, lemon yellow, cherry, lime, rose, lavender, orchid, violet, daffodil yellow, lilac, buttercup.

Consider, too, the butterflies—from orange and black to exotic blue-greens. And notice the spectrum at the seashore: the pink of the crabs, the stunning purple of the sea urchin, the pearlescent shades of an abalone shell.

See what an infinite variety of greens we have, beginning with the green of moss or new willow leaves or spring grass, deepening to the pine, then to the leaves of camellias and magnolias.

When I'm holding color training sessions for my consultants, I like to take them on a nature walk in the woods where they can experience some of these variations as well as the browns and grays of the tree trunks, the yellow of the mustard plant blossoms, and so much more.

Our Creator has also painted deserts, mountains, and prairies with lavish color, and has softened them all with the blues of the sky, lakes, and oceans.

He bestowed upon mammals dramatic contrasts in coloration: the brown-black and cream of the zebra, the red of the fox, gray of the squirrel, gold tones of a retriever, auburn of an Irish setter.

Does it sometimes seem to you that, compared to the color around us, man is a little "blah"? How can our limited variations of yellow, brown, red, and beige skin compare with the rest of his universe?

Well, perhaps we were created neutral in skin tones so we could be *receivers* of the glorious bounty of color God has created. Certainly he felt concern about color in our lives, for notice how he specified the colors of the priests' clothing in Exodus, calling for shades of gold, blue, purple, and scarlet.

He also gave us alone, in all creation, the privilege of choosing the colors of what we wear.

But with privilege comes responsibility. And in the case of color, that responsibility surely is to learn to choose wisely.

That is what we want to help you do in this chapter.

COLOR IMPACT

What a vast array of colors we have from which to choose today! At one time, color was restricted to the wealthy because of the great cost of the dyes. Later, less expensive synthetic dyes brought color to all classes. But the real "color revolution" came in the early 1960s, prompted by the advent of color TV. It changed our attitudes and preferences regarding color and brought hundreds of new colors into availability and popularity, in everything from household paints to men's shirts.

Have you ever thought about the tremendous impact color exerts in our lives today? It can stimulate or depress—actually changing our behavior.

Industry has learned this: The wrong colors in an office or factory can destroy employee morale, while the right colors can increase productivity. In one factory, workmen lifting black boxes complained that they were too heavy. When the cartons were painted green, they were sure they were lighter.

On the other hand, a French airline upholstered the interior of its planes in a yellow-green and noticed a sharp increase in the incidence of air sickness. Yet psychologists have found that a room painted a certain shade of pink has a quieting effect on people who are agitated or violent.

And why do you suppose fast food restaurants use bright, often jangling combinations of yellow, orange, and shocking pink? So we won't linger over our food. Other restaurants use red because it's stimulating, even to the appetite. Red, in fact, is a color which invariably captures attention. When I'm speaking, my eye naturally moves to the red sweaters and blouses in the audience. It's the color to wear when you're shopping and want to be waited on promptly. I recently recommended it to a client who came to us because she wished to be chosen from a number of applicants to appear on a TV game show. It works. But red cars also get more traffic tickets!

Actually, we assign a number of different, and sometimes contradictory meanings, to various colors.

Red is dominant, dynamic, energy raising, but also warlike. It can symbolize hate and anger as well as love, beauty, cheer. It is thought to be the first color perceived by babies; and children reach for it first to use in their coloring books.

Blue is considered cool, orderly, honest, and is associated with divinity, trust, loneliness, lovers, sadness, "the blues," infinity. The "people's color," it's the favorite choice in clothes for young people.

Purple is royal, creates distances, indicates sorrow, weariness, solemnity. Violet implies depth of feeling, spirituality. Lavender is feminine, delicate.

Yellow represents light, glory, cheer, wisdom, but also dual personality, cowardice, jealousy. Gold is associated with wealth.

Orange has virtually no negative association emotionally or culturally. It is cheerful, expansive, rich, and extroverted, although muddier shades can be irritating and "cheap." It has domestic qualities and is often used in the kitchen.

Brown, a darkened hue of orange, represents the shades of the earth. It is linked with comfort, mellowness, warmth, coziness.

Green is the color of life and health, indicates rebirth, the power of nature. It is the most restful color to the eye and may denote money to us. But it is also linked with nausea, poison, envy, and jealousy, and can be related to the weird—"green men from Mars."

White indicates hope, joy, innocence, virtue, purity, the sterile and clinical, as well as surrender. (It is also harsh in comparison with our own softer natural colors. Never wear a white which is whiter than your eyes or teeth, for it will make them appear yellow.)

Black is cold, somber, gloomy, mysterious, ominous, related to sorrow. Most of our associations with it are negative except for our image of it as glamorous.

Color also prompts value judgments from others. Gray and navy blue, for instance, are considered businesslike by most people and also tend to denote affluence. Neutrals are nonthreatening and soothing. A speaker would do well to wear a neutral, because it is not tiring to the eyes and does not distract from the content of the message.

THE 12-SEASON COLOR SYSTEM™

Color, as a designer recently noted, "is so important today in every part of our lives. It's the number one factor in attracting the customer to any product."

The most important aspect of color for you to understand, however, is that all shades of all colors are not suited to each of us.

My study of color indicates that there are certain colors which are in harmony with each person, and others which are not. And, just as God created us as unique persons in terms of style and body types, he has also created us with our own unique color patterns which give us distinction and set each of us apart as an individual.

Have you noticed how the foliage on each plant is designed to enhance its flower? The green is always just the right shade to harmonize with and enrich the color of the blossom. So, too, certain colors will make your skin appear smooth, clear, and glowing, minimize lines and circles, and generate a healthy glow. When you wear "your" colors, you feel at home in God's universe.

Our clues to the "right" colors come directly from that universe. For God paints with a different palette of colors each season of the year. Notice what fresh, clear colors he uses in the spring, when all is cleansed by melted snow and early rains. There's a sparkling awakening about spring, a rich oneness, no matter how many colors delight our eyes. Daffodils, tulips, crocuses—they're all bright and new, all reflections of sunlight.

Then, as the sun moves higher in the sky, its summer intensity seems to quiet the hues. Flowers become more muted, as though washed with a soft blue; or, later in the season, with a bit of gray. Twilights streak with rose and the heat of summer seems to modulate, soften, tone down the colors around us.

With fall, nature turns flamboyant once again, with the yellows, oranges, reds, and bronzes of the changing leaves, the rich shades of chrysanthemums. Colors glow rich and mellow, warm as the fires we begin to light in our fireplaces.

In winter, nature rests, and the world turns black and white and gray. Inside, we warm ourselves with clear primary colors, such as the dramatic accent of poinsettias. Outside, icy colors with cool blue undertones prevail. It's our season of strongest contrasts.

Everyone has personal coloring—in the skin, the eyes, the hair—which is in harmony with a particular portion of one of these seasons. Perhaps you're already familiar with the seasonal color theory, which is being applied more and more today in helping women find their most becoming colors. Actually, it was inspired by the study of artist and colorist Johannes Itten of Germany. He discovered the power of personal coloring in directing a student's choice of colors in his paintings. Itten noted that a student's personal colors were consistently those complementary to his skin tones, hair, and eyes, in both tone and intensity.

The most important key to the season with which your coloring is compatible is your basic skin tone. This is not always easy to determine. But if you look at the skin on the inside of your wrist, you may be able to tell whether the undertones are gold (spring or fall), or if they tend to be blue with a pinkish cast (summer or winter). If you're not sure, try viewing your inner wrist against pure white fabric or paper, or compare it with others'.

Sometimes it's enlightening to squeeze one of your fingers near its tip. Notice, as its color deepens, whether the tone is more yellow-red (spring or fall) or blue-red (summer or winter). The best test, however, is draping yourself in different colored fabrics. We'll explain this later in the chapter.

First, let's take an overall look at the seasons of color.

Spring. The spring person has gold skin tones, but may vary from pale ivory to pink or peach to medium beige. Sometimes she is freckled, but she may be either very fair or easily tanned. She is often of Scandinavian heritage, or her ancestors may come from the British Isles, the Netherlands, or northern Europe.

Spring's hair varies from flaxen blonde to golden honey, strawberry blonde or light to medium brown with golden highlights. Many springs were blonde as children, and their hair darkens as they mature. It grays with a yellowish cast.

Eyes may be sparkling blue, blue-green, aqua, brown, gray-green, topaz. Often, they have golden flecks (which you can see with a magnifying mirror).

The spring palette blossoms in clear, delicate colors with warm yellow undertones.

Summer. The summer woman has rosy, delicate skin tones, ranging from the very pale to a deeper rose-beige. She can usually trace her lineage to northern Europe, the British Isles, Scandinavian countries, the Netherlands. Hair gleams ash blonde or may be soft brown, grayish brown, or possibly black. It grays with a silver tone. Eyes shine clear blue or misty blue, violet or hazel, and flecks are usually white. Summer identifies with the pastels of June and the soft colors of sea and sky, with their cool, blue undertones.

Autumn. The autumn person's skin is warm-toned with gold undertones, ranging from very fair ivory, to peach, to a ruddy, bronze cast. She may be freckled. She can be a blend of many backgrounds, although the redheaded Irish colleen is definitely an autumn.

Hair varies from bronze to red-brown, copper, medium brown, or tawny, and often has red highlights. It grays with a yellowish tone. Eyes are green, gray-green, topaz, olive, yellow-green with gold flecks, red-brown, blue-green, or brown. Autumn's color palette radiates in the warm, rich colors of fall, with their golden undertones.

Winter. Winter's skin will have blue undertones with a purple base and can be black, brown, red-brown, olive, or light. Light to dark olive are the most common, and they can be confusing to judge because the blue undertone may not show through (since the skin is often thick and may look yellow). Sometimes the blue undertone combined with the yellow overtone can give a gray effect.

Her origins are tremendously varied: dark Irish, Welsh, southern European, South American, American Indian, Polynesian, East Asian, East Indian. Most Blacks, Hispanics, and Orientals are winters. There are, in fact, more winters in the world than the other seasons.

Hair may be black, dark brown, silver gray (not golden gray), or white, and eyes are usually gray, gray-green, gray-blue, black, or brown. The winter palette sparkles in the vivid, clear primary colors and cool, icy colors with blue undertones.

As you can see, there is a tremendous and confusing variety within each of these seasons. And the more I've worked with color palettes, the more I realize that only 50 percent of the women have skin, eye, and hair coloring which is in harmony with the classic, traditional perception of these seasons.

For the rest, some of the colors in their supposed season looked wonderful; others were either too pale or too overpowering. Gradually, I began to realize that there are actually twelve groupings, not just four. And when I began to subdivide them into the months of the year, I found that virtually everyone could be accommodated.

It has been so gratifying to see how this new system clarifies and relieves the confusion and frustration so many women have felt about their palettes when they were typed simply as spring, summer, fall, or winter. Turn to the color pages of this book and you will begin to see how the 12-Season Color System™ works.

(Note that we've specified the months of each season to be best in harmony with nature's change around us, not to coincide with the calendar.)

As you look at the different palettes, can you see why it's so difficult to fit women into just four seasons?

Here are just a few of the women who had "aha!" experiences as they learned which month they fit into.

An airline stewardess, a radiant gold blonde with deep tan skin, was disappointed in the classic spring palette, because she loved bright, strong colors. (She really wanted to be a winter.) Now, however, she is totally pleased with the lovely vivid colors of her March palette (bright spring).

Lynda had been classified as a summer, and was truly faithful to the palette she'd been given, often wearing blue undertone pinks and raspberry—which her husband hated. When she came in to train with us as a consultant, she saw that she was warm but not bright, and too light to be a gentle autumn. The soft, muted colors of May, the gentle spring, are exactly right for her.

However, another woman couldn't understand why the soft, muted summer colors didn't do a thing for her. "This is the best day of my life!" she declared, when she discovered how radiant she is in the clearer colors which suit her perfectly as a June—a bright summer.

A soft personality often goes hand-in-hand with the August, gentle summer palette. This was true for one client, who felt overwhelmed by the brights and deeper tones of the classic summer. She was pleased to find the soft, dusty colors which complement her personality, and is superb in anything with a soft violet wash.

Carol, on the other hand, felt drab in the muted colors she'd been given when she was judged to be an autumn. Her flaming red hair and peach skin demand colors with clear, light, warm undertones. Her dark hair is not as bright as a bright spring, or as muted as a classic autumn. She is a true September: bright autumn.

However, the colors which are fabulous on Carol drained all the color from Ann's face. When she tried to wear a bright red sweater (a shade she'd been given in her autumn palette), her face grew so pale, she tried to add more and more blusher—achieving only the effect of two bright slashes of color on her cheeks. Intense green was also overpowering to her. Now that she understands she's a November, a gentle autumn, she loves the soft, muted tones which are so definitely hers.

As for the December, or bright winter, we've found that our brightest color swatches remain in our boxes. Occasionally a woman with white hair, a black girl, or a "Snow White" (light skin and dark hair) comes along and looks radiant in these shades. But we were never able to give them to what we now realize is the classic winter woman, the January. She is best in the medium brights. And certainly these super brights overwhelmed the gentle winter, the February.

Most winters, we find, are Februarys, and they are distressed when they receive the bright shades of a prepackaged winter palette. Susan, a quiet, elegant woman, was horrified at the powerful colors she was given, and vastly relieved when she learned she is a gentle February.

How are you feeling at this point? Confused? Overwhelmed? Doubtful? That it may not be worth the effort to determine your own palette?

I want to encourage you to persevere. I truly believe you will be as excited about your "right" colors as my clients are. If the concept of the different seasons is familiar to you, I hope the breakdown of the months within the season has helped clarify the complexities of color for you.

If all this is brand new to you, do take the time to read and reread it. Then, see if you can find out which month you are. If you're not certain, enlist the aid of your family or friends.

Remove your makeup. If you color your hair to a shade very different from its natural tint, be sure to cover it, since hair color can actually change the appearance of your skin tone.

Now, using a white sheet over your clothes to block out other colors, try draping your shoulder and neck area with various colors. If you can find a piece of shiny gold material and a piece of shiny silver, you and your friends should very quickly see which is more becoming. If it's the gold, you are probably a spring or fall. To determine which, see whether a soft gold (spring) or a rich amber gold (fall) does the most for your skin, eyes, and hair.

If the silver fabric is more becoming than the gold, you are most likely a winter or summer. To help you decide which, try draping yourself with burgundy and with dusty rose. If the burgundy is most becoming, you are probably a winter; but if the rose is better, you are a summer.

If you're still having difficulty deciding, here are some additional tests:

Summer vs. Spring
Off-white vs. cream
Dusty rose vs. peach
Pink vs. soft gold

Winter vs. Autumn
Burgundy vs. rust
Black vs. brown
Blue-green vs. avocado

If you've colored your hair, you can also use wigs to help you determine your season:

gold brown vs. ash brown: autumn vs. winter
golden blonde vs. silver blonde: spring vs. summer

Let me caution you about a few factors which could affect your decision. Illness and medications can affect your skin color. So, too, a deep tan can sometimes confuse you, since it does enable you to wear brighter colors. And aging skin sometimes tends to turn light olive with a yellowish cast, which could be confused with golden undertones.

Also, some people find it difficult to distinguish between the olive skin which is common to winter and the golden tones of autumn and spring. Olive skins actually have a blue undertone with a purple base, but there is a yellow overtone which produces the confusion.

The best test is to try yellow-undertoned colors (yellow-green, orange-yellow-red), then colors with blue undertones (blue-green and blue-red). If the yellow makes the skin look very yellow and tired, but the blue brings up the rosiness, giving a healthy, vibrant look, you are dealing with the olive skin of a winter, not the golden skin of a spring or autumn.

FINDING YOUR MONTH

As for which month you are within a given season, take a close look at the intensity of your own coloring. The lighter and brighter you look, the more likely you are to be a "bright." If you have medium intensity, you are probably a classic. But if your coloring is very soft, you are a gentle palette.

If you're still not certain, try different intensities of color. For instance, if you feel you are a spring, see if a bright tomato red makes you look vibrant. If it does, you are a bright spring, a March. If, however, a softer, more subdued red is more becoming, you are probably a classic spring, an April. But if a pale peach brings life to your skin, while the bright red washes you out, you are probably a gentle spring, a May.

One excellent test of whether you're wearing your best colors is other people's comments. If they tell you, "What a beautiful dress," or, "That's a gorgeous color," be careful. If they say, "How wonderful you look!" it's a good indication you're wearing a color that is uniquely yours.

Incidentally, women sometimes ask me why they receive compliments when they wear a color which is not in their palette. Sometimes, we've found, it's because the observer loves that particular color, or because of the style of the dress. Other times, the observer is actually complimenting the change or the newness of what's being worn, rather than the effect of the color upon the woman.

Pay close attention, too, to how you *feel* in various colors. You have more innate sense of color than you may think you do!

If you're confused about your palette, or would like confirmation of your decision, by all means write to us. Use the coupon in the back of the book for your own personal color palette from Uniquely You.

How to combine your colors. There is still another dimension to using color.

Not only do you have certain colors which are most becoming

to you; you also have certain color *combinations* which are most flattering.

If you have gentle contrasts in your own personal coloring (for instance, medium brown hair and medium beige skin), you will look best in gently contrasting colors.

However, if your personal coloring is in strong contrast (such as ivory skin and black hair), you can effectively wear much stronger contrasts in colors. Indeed, the gentle contrasts will be overwhelming to you.

To help you understand these combinations, let me first define our color terms.

Soft dark: a gentle shade, such as a soft, dark navy
Soft light: also gentle, as a soft, light pink
Medium: a color which is not really dark and not really light; in the middle, in terms of intensity (rose is an example)
Dark: a color with black added, such as a dark navy
Light: a color with a lot of white added, such as light pink
Pastel: a shade between medium and light—a pastel pink would not be as pale as a light pink
Bright: a color which is strong in saturation, loaded with color, and contains less black or white; bright red
Blended Medium: two shades of the same value; neither light nor dark, such as lavender or rose
Muted pastel: a grayed, toned-down shade, such as cloud gray

Now here are some guidelines on how to combine colors within your palette.

COMBINING COLORS WITHIN YOUR OWN PALETTE.
March (bright spring) and April (classic spring) wear light-bright combinations:
soft dark/soft light, dark/light, bright/light, bright/bright, 1 light, 1 bright. Avoid: blended medium, 1 muted pastel, dark/bright, dark/dark.

May (gentle spring) wears gentle combinations:
soft dark/soft light, blended medium, medium/dark, medium/light, pastel/pastel, light/medium/dark, 1 medium. Avoid: dark/light, light/bright, dark/bright, bright/bright.

June (bright summer) wears light-bright combinations:
soft dark/soft light, dark/light, bright/light, bright/bright, 1 light, 1 bright, blended medium. Avoid: 1 muted pastel, dark/bright, dark/dark.

July (classic summer) and August (gentle summer) wear gentle combinations:
soft dark/soft light, blended medium, medium/dark, medium/light, pastel/pastel, light/medium/dark, 1 medium. Avoid: dark/light, light/bright, dark/bright, bright/bright.

September (bright autumn) wears light-bright combinations:
soft dark/soft light, dark/light, bright/light, bright/bright, 1 light, 1 bright, dark/bright. Avoid: blended medium, 1 muted pastel, dark/dark.

October (classic autumn) wears muted combinations:
soft dark/soft light, blended medium, medium/light, medium/dark, light/medium/dark, 1 medium, 1 dark. Avoid: dark/light, pastel/pastel, 1 pastel, bright/bright, light/bright.

November (gentle autumn) wears gentle combinations:
soft dark/soft light, blended medium, medium/dark, medium/light, pastel/pastel, light/medium/dark, 1 medium. Avoid: dark/light, light/bright, dark/bright, bright/bright.

December, January, February (winter palettes) wear contrast:
dark/light, dark/bright, light/bright, bright/bright, 1 bright. Avoid: light/light, blended medium, dark/dark, 1 light, 1 dark.

It is so exciting for me to see women who have looked dull and lifeless begin literally to glow, to receive compliments at club meetings or at work, when they start wearing their best colors.

When Connie came to me, she had tried every hair color on the shelf. More recently she had used henna, which reflected on her skin, giving a harsh, ruddy tone. Today her hair is its natural brunette shade, and she is gorgeous in her rich, classic winter colors.

Another woman had tinted her hair a golden blonde, which also reflected and made her skin look golden. She appeared to be a spring. But when we covered her hair and tested various colors, we found that she was a summer—a July. Now her hair is ash blonde and she looks smashing in her cool, muted colors.

Still another had her color analyzed four times elsewhere. Half her palettes were spring, half summer. We found her skin to be pink-beige, but with pigmentation changes from taking birth control pills, which gave her a gold cast. She is a light, bright summer, a June, with a small palette to compensate for the pigmentation. We cautioned her against dark neutrals and urged her to use light, bright, cool undertone colors. Teal, raspberry, medium blue, blue-green, and pale yellow all clarify her skin.

My co-author, Bev, was a puzzlement at first. Two different people had classified her as an autumn, and she did have freckles, the red highlights to the hair, and a golden look to her skin which would be associated with an autumn. But her hair was beginning to gray in a true silver gray, not a yellowed gray. And as we worked together and I saw her in her camel jacket and rust print blouse, I began to wonder. So we removed her makeup and tested her under a white light. When we draped her with both a gold lamé and a silver lamé, there was little question. The gold turned her yellow, while the silver made her skin clear and her blue eyes sparkle. We thought at first she might be a summer, but as we held the various colors to her, it became clear that she is a soft, gentle winter—a February. The olive tones of her skin had been mistaken for the gold tones of autumn.

I had a similar experience because my skin also tends to light olive. So I first thought I was a spring. Actually, I'm a light, bright summer—a June. I wear brighter colors with blue undertones and have a limited palette. My best colors: off-white, raspberry, blue-red, medium and navy blue, periwinkle blue, blue-green, pale yellow.

Bev looked OK in her fall shades, but she is radiant in her bright blues, navys, and blue-reds. Interesting, these were the very colors she could not bring herself to give away when she cleaned her closet. She was relieved to learn that she had a better eye than she'd thought! And while she disliked many of the colors in her old autumn palette, she loves every color in her new palette.

Incidentally, because of her olive overtones, she cannot wear certain shades of pink and wine which other winters wear well; they cause her to appear more yellow.

This is why I never give out "pre-fab" colors. ("You're a summer; here's your palette.") Each person *is* unique. I still find that, depending on her natural coloring, a woman may wear fifty to seventy-five or more colors well. If she has changed her natural coloring by tinting her hair or wearing contact lenses, she may reduce her colors to as few as twenty. I feel it's vital to do each palette individually.

One of the great bonuses of understanding your best colors is that it greatly simplifies your shopping. At a sale, you can simply glance down the clothes on the rack till you come to a color which is one of yours. You'll save literally hours of shopping.

One word of caution, however: always check colors in natural light. Many's the color mistake I've made which stemmed from a store's deceptive lighting.

Knowing your colors will also save you from buying a color just because it's in fashion this season. A beautiful classic winter woman came to me recently wearing khaki. She'd bought it when it was in all the stores, but she looked like a tired candidate for the army reserve. It drained her so, I couldn't wait to show her the wonderful jewel tones which would be so becoming.

MOVING INTO YOUR BEST COLORS

But what about all the clothes in your closet today which now seem "wrong" in color? You're not quite ready to toss them all out? Go at it gradually. Give the worst offenders to a friend for whom the color is right. Bev recently loaned a wine velvet jacket (which turned her skin yellow) to a silver-haired classic winter friend. When Bev saw how beautiful her friend looked, she knew she had to give the jacket to her. What a pleasure to see her enjoying it!

Many of my consultants have had fun exchanging clothing. What's "wrong" for you may be exactly right for someone else.

Also, while you're gravitating toward your best colors, you might continue to wear your not-so-best colors, but keep them away from your face. If, for instance, you realize your black suit is harsh and unflattering, wear the skirt or pants with a top which is in one of your best colors.

Consider it a five-year plan to buy gradually into your own palette. And each time you bring home something new, make it a point to give something away. This was difficult for me until I read Anne Ortlund's *Disciplines of the Beautiful Woman.* In it, she pleads, "Oh, women! It is just wicked to cram and stuff our closets and drawers with things we seldom wear or don't need to wear! Continually get rid of them. Keep giving and giving! . . . Keep stripped down. In your wardrobe as well as in the rest of your life, 'eliminate and concentrate.'"

Now that you are beginning to recognize your palette, you can use color within it in subtle ways. Neutrals (beige, gray, oyster) are perhaps best when you wish the other person to feel more secure, when it's important not to overwhelm or set up competition. There is great serenity in lack of color; note the beauty of a moonlit night which gives the feeling of walking through a black and white movie.

However, if you wish to be noticed and to attract others to you, you may want to choose a more vivid color from your palette. Red is the most obvious, but turquoise, electric blue, yellow, or orange are equally eye-catching.

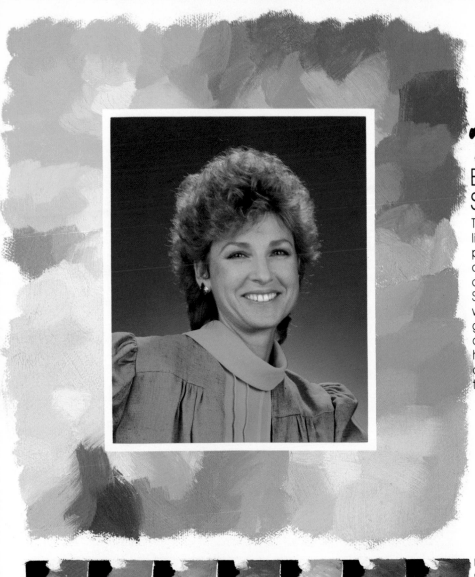

march

BRIGHT SPRING

The bright spring is very light and bright in appearance. She carries all the clear bright and contrasting light colors. She is different from the winter because of her golden undertone coloring. The red-black hair type can wear clear, dark, warm neutrals.

EYES: clear green, clear blue, aqua, French blue, light blue, olive with orange flecks, light golden brown

HAIR: light golden blonde, warm white, flaxen blonde, strawberry redhead, red-black, brown-black

SKIN: ivory, fair ivory, deep peach, rosy glow, dark olive with yellow base

April

CLASSIC SPRING

The classic spring has a light, bright appearance that is not as vivid as the bright spring. She wears medium light, bright colors that are clear but not overwhelming. She looks good in contrast, but should avoid the darks.

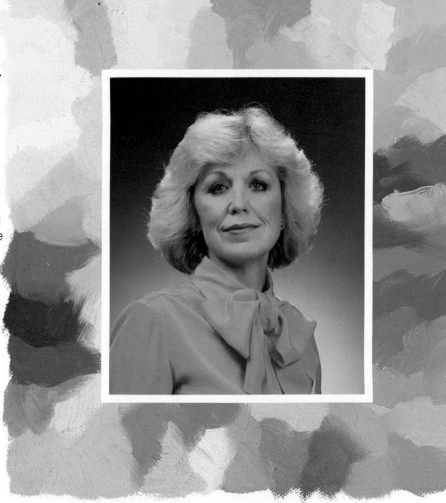

EYES: blue-gray, golden brown, blue-green, light brown, aqua

HAIR: golden blonde, light warm brown, golden gray, yellow-brown chestnut, strawberry blonde

SKIN: warm beige, pale beige, fair peach, ivory, peach-pink, peach

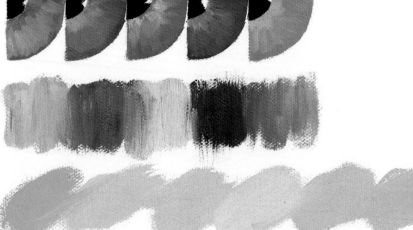

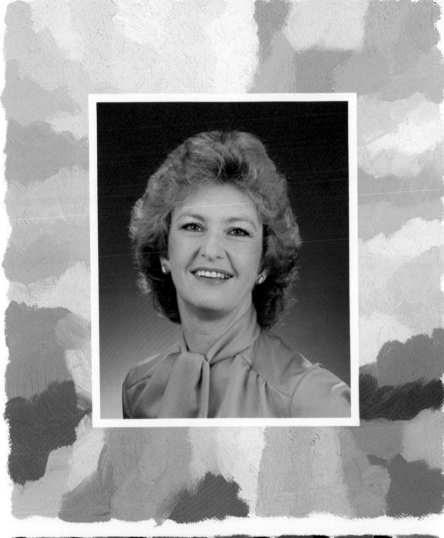

may

GENTLE SPRING

The gentle spring has a very soft, light, muted appearance. She is too light to wear the deeper muted colors of autumn and cannot carry the clear brights of spring.

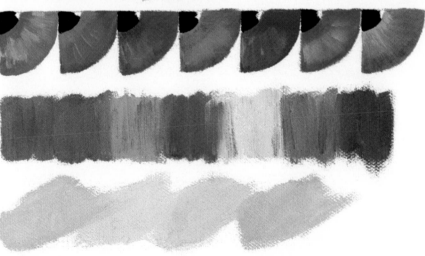

EYES: blue-green, gray-green, hazel, topaz, green-brown, steel gray, soft golden brown

HAIR: soft honey blonde, soft strawberry blonde, sandy red, medium dishwater blonde, light yellow-gray, light amber

SKIN: light golden beige, pale ivory, peach-ivory, beige

June

BRIGHT SUMMER

The overall appearance of the bright summer is light and bright, yet she is not a spring, but has the cool undertone coloring. She wears the clearer summer colors and should avoid the dark, very drab, muted colors.

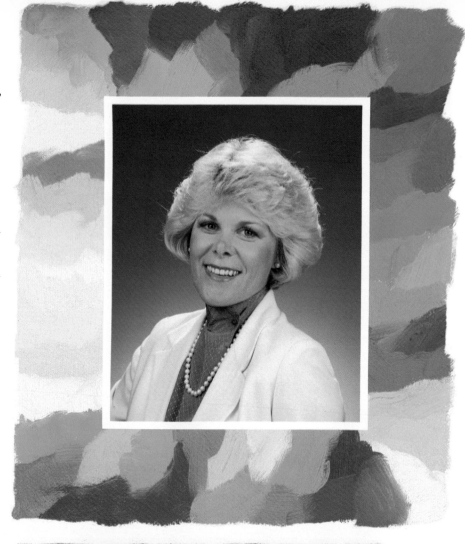

EYES: pale aqua, deep blue, blue-gray, blue-green, blue, or green

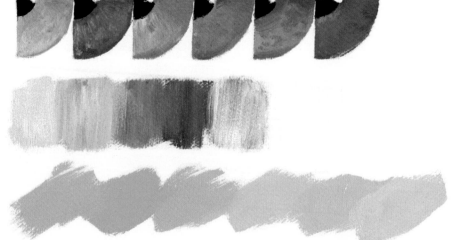

HAIR: light ash blonde, ash with silver gray highlights, medium ash blonde, light ash blonde with golden highlights, light silver gray

SKIN: beige, very pink, deep rose beige, light rose beige, medium olive, light olive

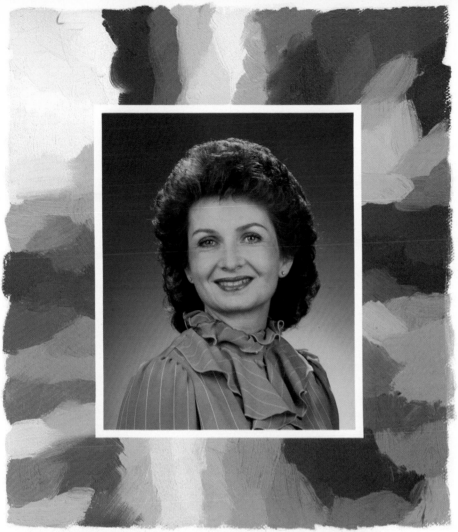

July

CLASSIC SUMMER

The classic summer has a soft, cool appearance. Her colors range from gentle brights to muted blue undertones. She can wear soft-dark contrasts, and favors blended colors in medium tones.

EYES: blue, gray-blue, hazel, gray-green, gray, gray-brown

HAIR: blonde, medium brown with auburn cast, blue-gray, dark ash blonde, silver gray, gray-brown, medium/dark ash brown, medium brown

SKIN: rose beige, beige, pink-beige, violet-ivory

august

GENTLE SUMMER

The gentle summer has almost an all-one-color appearance. She is the gentlest of all the palettes. Her colors are extremely soft, dusty, and muted, from a middle to light range. Darks are overpowering unless combined with a middle or light value.

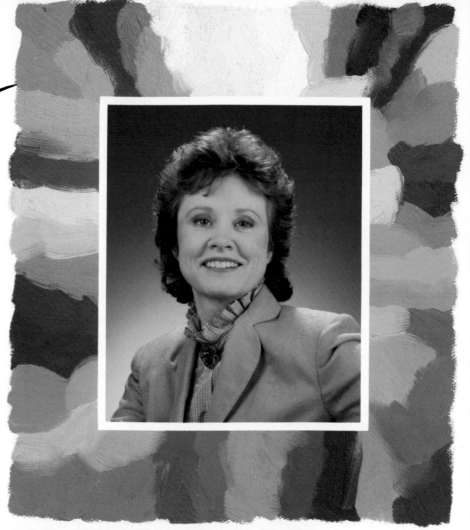

EYES: blue-gray, gray-green, pale gray, brown, hazel

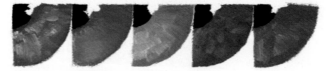

HAIR: medium ash blonde, light ash brown, soft silver gray, medium charcoal gray-brown

SKIN: pale beige, delicate pink cheeks, fair, delicate pink, violet-gray cast over ivory or pink

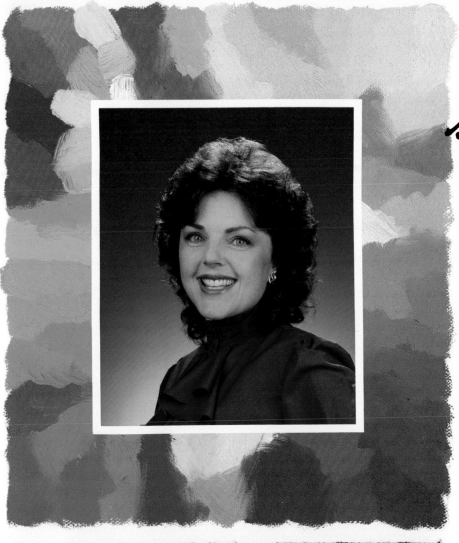

September

BRIGHT AUTUMN

The bright autumn is comparable to the winter palette; because she wears clearer, brighter autumn colors, and in contrast. The classic autumn muted colors are dull and not in harmony with this bright coloring. Her colors have golden undertones.

EYES: aquamarine, dark/medium gold-brown, avocado green, green cat eyes, turquoise, light reddish brown, rust brown, olive green

HAIR: coppery red-brown, light pewter, bright red, gold with red highlights, deep auburn, brown-black, chestnut brown, golden black, golden blonde

SKIN: golden black, florid, light peach, dark copper beige, dark beige, light yellow beige, ivory

October
CLASSIC AUTUMN

The classic autumn wears the deep, rich, muted earth tones. Her overall coloring is gentle and softened, with medium to dark colors. She must avoid clear and strong, bright colors.

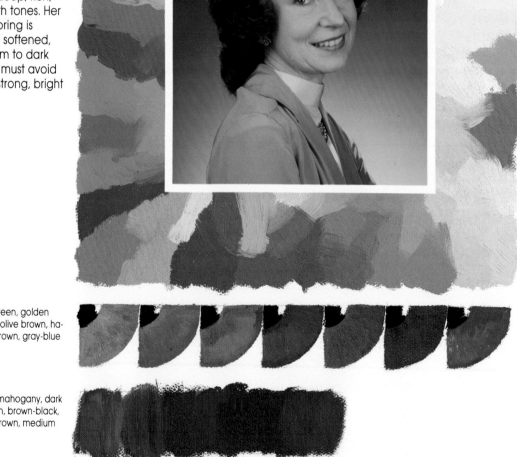

EYES: yellow, green, golden amber brown, olive brown, hazel, dark red-brown, gray-blue

HAIR: auburn, mahogany, dark chestnut brown, brown-black, dark golden brown, medium brown

SKIN: light brown, bronze, deep peach, golden beige, medium yellow beige, ivory

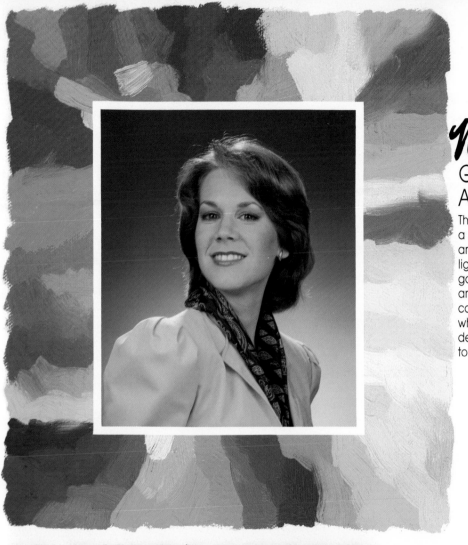

November

GENTLE AUTUMN

The gentle autumn, has a soft overall appearance. She wears the lighter muted tones, golden undertones, and blended medium colors. She is overwhelmed in the deeper, darker muted tones.

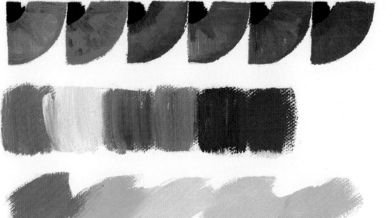

EYES: topaz, pale misty green, light golden brown, light rust-brown, hazel, hazel brown

HAIR: light golden brown, golden gray, medium golden brown, dark strawberry blonde, medium brown

SKIN: soft yellow-brown, peach beige, ivory with golden freckles, soft yellow beige, soft golden

December

BRIGHT WINTER

The bright winter has the strongest, brightest coloring of all palettes. She is radiant in contrast, using dark and light, and is especially good in brights alone or combinations.

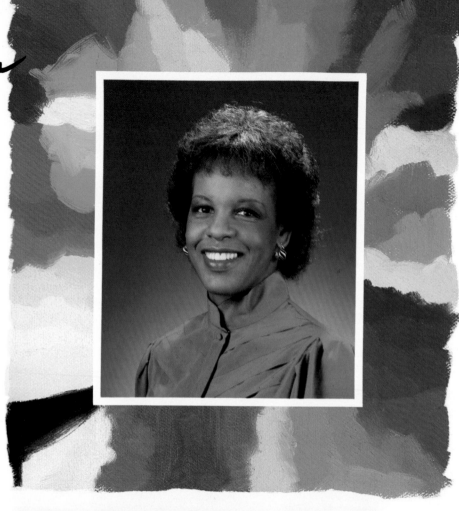

EYES: dark red-brown, black-brown, green, turquoise, brown, blue-violet

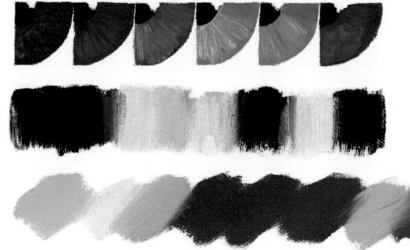

HAIR: black, blue-black, oyster white, white-blonde, white, silver gray, dark chestnut black, platinum blonde, gray-black

SKIN: light rose beige, white-alabaster, dark olive, black, brown-black, brown, pink-peach, red-brown

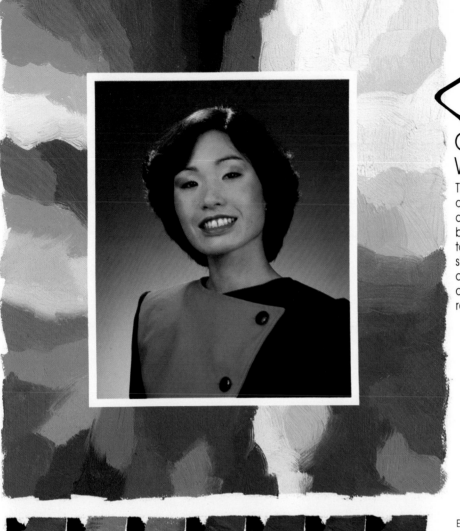

January

CLASSIC WINTER

The classic winter wears all the beautiful medium-bright, clear hues, but is overwhelmed by too strong or vivid shades. She carries contrast well and wears a light to very dark range.

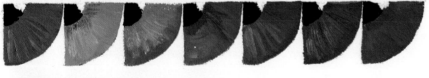

EYES: gray blue, light blue, blue with white flecks, dark blue, golden brown, olive brown, pine green, brown with yellow highlights

HAIR: brown-black walnut, chestnut brown, salt and pepper, light silver gray

SKIN: light olive, beige, white, delicate pink tone, medium rose beige, champagne beige, olive, yellow-brown

February

GENTLE WINTER

The gentle winter is darker in appearance than the summer but wears muted winter colors that have a soft look. She is overwhelmed in the strong, clear brights of winter.

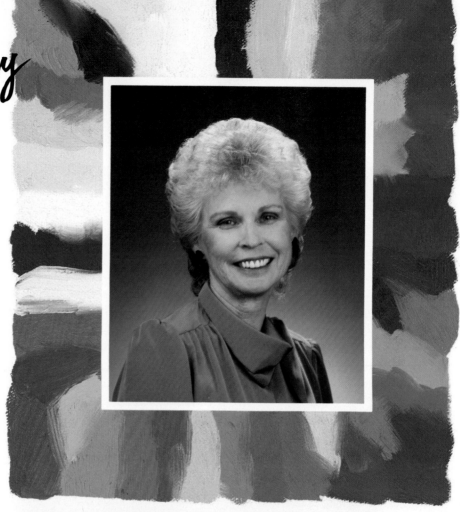

EYES: hazel, gray-blue, gray-green, light brown, olive brown, dark blue

HAIR: dark ash brown, dark/medium brown, light charcoal gray

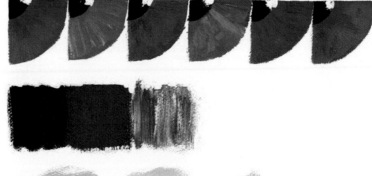

SKIN: rose beige, champagne beige, light olive

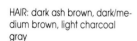

Look back over the earlier part of this chapter and refresh your memory as to what colors give out which messages to others.

Women frequently ask me, "What if I absolutely adore a color which isn't at all mine?"

Use it in decorating. Enjoy looking at it, but avoid wearing it. If it's already a large part of your wardrobe and you can't yet bear to part with it, relieve it with blouses or scarves in colors which truly flatter you.

Other often-asked questions: "Will my palette change as I grow older, grayer?" (No, but we do soften with age. See details in hair chapter.) "What happens as I tan?" (Your palette is the same, but you may wear brighter shades.)

As you start to understand the harmony of God's color plan, you'll develop an awareness of those around you. You'll begin to understand why some people have such a glow, such clarity of skin, why their hair shines more and their eyes sparkle. And you'll wish you could tactfully say something to that girl with the smashing red hair who insists upon wearing lavender, or the dramatic woman with the blue-black hair whose mustard-colored blouse turns her face a sickly sallow. And maybe, gently, you can. (You might pass this book along to them!)

But please, don't be an oh-yes-I've-had-my-colors-done-and-I-wear-what-I-like person. Don't be swayed by "the" colors of the year as prescribed by designers and fashion "authorities."

Perhaps you're feeling questioning or uneasy about this matter of "your" colors. But I think you'll find, as so many, many women have, that understanding and using your best colors, realizing, "I'm a January," is not pigeon-holing or putting yourself in a box. Instead, it is truly freeing.

I'd encourage you to learn the lessons of God's earth cycle. Work with the color clues God has given you, not against them. Appropriate his color plan so that your apparel becomes a reflection of the truth about you, without artificiality or distortion. The more authentic you seem, the more you will be able to give to others.

Join in the harmony of God's universe. You *will* be beautiful!

BEAUTY IS CONTRAST

MALE AND FEMALE HE CREATED US

In working with hundreds of women each month, I seem to hear again and again about their difficulties with their husbands or the "meaningful males" in their lives. The men, they tell me, just "don't understand" them. And it seems to me that at least 80 percent of the time the problem is rooted in the failure of the woman (and sometimes the man) to understand the male/female differences or contrasts, and to accept them.

For instance, one woman told how her husband found one reason after another not to finish planting the many bushes and trees which waited in plastic pots for the landscaping of their new home. Finally, angry and impatient, she decided she'd do it—and better. She spent a whole weekend, while he was out of town, planting six bushes. It was hard, hot work in clay and shale soil. So when he came home and saw what she had done and failed to praise her, she was *furious!* She couldn't understand why he didn't appreciate all her labor. She wanted him to apologize for not doing it himself.

Another woman, a club-champion caliber tennis player, was baffled that her husband, a mediocre player, refused ever to team up with her for doubles. "I'd love to do this together with him. He just doesn't seem to realize how much it would mean to me."

It appears to me that both these women, failing to understand their female nature, have placed themselves in competition with their husbands' basic need to excel in performance.

Do you, also, see many marriages around you today which are locked in no-win power struggles? Perhaps it's because more and more women are in the competitive job market and find it difficult to stop jockeying for position when they come home. Perhaps it's because the women's movement has distorted some people's thinking till they see men and women as being exactly alike, of the same nature.

The woman who planted the bushes, in trying to do it better than her husband, was really competing with him, or trying to be "the same."

Surely this isn't God's intention for us. After all, "At the beginning the Creator 'made them male and female' " (Matthew 19:4).

In Genesis 2:18, we learn how, after God first created man in his own image, he saw that something was missing.

That was when he created woman. Woman, not another man! Woman, a contrast. And Adam's ecstatic reaction was, "At last!" ("This at last is bone of my bones and flesh of my flesh," Genesis 2:24, RSV).

Would he have responded so enthusiastically if God had created someone just like him? I doubt it.

It seems to me that if we want to sustain the "At last!" attitude in the men in our lives, if we want them to perceive us as beautiful, not just when we're twenty-one, but also when we're sixty-one, we need to remember the importance of maintaining this contrast.

God has equipped us to do this by building into each of us certain characteristics which are widely documented by psychologists. Men, for instance, tend to be more aggressive, dominant, logical, independent, active, ambitious, and task-oriented.

Women, on the other hand, are more likely to be intuitive, dependent, nurturant, supportive, patient, and person-oriented.

Now, of course, there is tremendous variation between individual men and women. (Yes, men can be intuitive and women logical.) But between most men and most women, the contrast will remain. And interestingly, anthropologists have confirmed that in societies where male-female roles are most clearly defined and contrasted, there is the most freedom for cross-overs in roles, perhaps because men and women are more secure with their sexual worth and can afford the risks.

I find that I "cross over" in my career in Uniquely You, where I function as a producer-achiever. But I learned long ago that I must remove that "hat" at home, and I am really very grateful to be able to do so. So I try to tell my husband how much I appreciate his chopping down the tree and sharing some responsibilities at home (he's a fantastic soup chef!) and doing productive things when he could have watched TV over the weekend. As I thank him for his ability to perform both at work and at home, he inevitably responds with concern for me and how I am *feeling*.

And isn't that what we really want from our men—for them to be sensitive to our feelings? They will be, if we recognize their ability to achieve specific tasks successfully.

In teaching Bible studies in southern California on male-female roles in marriage, Patricia DeVorss confirms my observations about the need to maintain the contrast between men and women. She finds that many women don't understand how important it is to a man's self-esteem for him to fulfill his role as the active, task-oriented provider-protector. And so, without realizing it, women may undermine their husbands by competing with them.

This is particularly true when a woman steps in to do a task a man is already working on, implying that she is better at it than he.

(The woman who planted the bushes accomplished her task efficiently. But in doing so, she did not allow her husband to function as provider-protector for her—to finish his task. And then, having diminished him as a man, she wondered why he didn't feel loving toward her and praise her!)

Especially in today's society, where roles have become blurred and even "exchanged," DeVorss feels God called woman to be a "helper" to her husband, to build up his masculinity and allow him his space to function as a male.

When she allows this, DeVorss observes, the man can cease his desperate struggle to be dominant and is then freed to be more caring and tender toward the woman, something most of us long for.

My co-author, Bev, gives an excellent example. A few days before Thanksgiving, she began feeling the pressure of a family holiday dinner to prepare, a sixtieth anniversary party to plan for her parents on December nineteenth, a church women's retreat to organize for early winter, Christmas shopping, Christmas cards—and a January 10 deadline for this book!

"I'm panicked," she admitted to her husband, Bob. "And I really need you. I don't mean to *do* things, but to help me stay focused and to support me in resisting other demands on my time."

That evening they had dinner at a casual little restaurant, and he said, "I think you should have the cake made for the folks' anniversary. And let the boys handle the Christmas tree and house decorations. And suspend all bread-baking for the duration."

"Wonderful!" she agreed.

They were quiet for a moment, and then he said, "You look just great tonight. In fact, you're the best-looking woman in this restaurant."

In Bev's eyes, she wasn't at all. But what mattered was that she was to her husband. For the truth is, when we allow a man to be a man, he perceives us differently. He actually sees us as beautiful from within.

And we in turn feel, and become, more beautiful.

GOD NEVER MENTIONED UNISEX

Certainly the muddying of male-female roles is reflected in many people's outward appearance today. Men wear gold chains, bracelets, and even earrings, as well as colors which once were considered feminine—such as pink and lilac. Women wear pants and sometimes don't bother shaving their legs. (Waiting outside the women's room at a theater recently, I heard a woman, mistaking a short-haired girl in T-shirt and blue jeans for a boy, tell her, "You're in the wrong line.") Today males and females emerge from the same salons with identical perms and haircuts.

Life gets confusing!

In Deuteronomy 22:5, God decrees, "A woman must not wear men's clothing, nor a man wear women's clothing."

As we live in the freedom of the New Testament, we know that Christ's death released us from the condemnation of those laws. Still, they remain signposts of God's desire that our dress reflect the differences of the male and female which he created.

And I think, deep down, this is our desire. Despite our love of wearing what's comfortable and functional, most of us would vastly prefer to look like women. Moreover, note that the song lyrics, "Why can't a woman be more like man?" do not ask, "Why can't a woman *look* more like a man?" (Remember in chapter 1, we saw how strongly men react to visual stimuli.)

As women, we need to ask ourselves, "Does my outer person mirror contentment with having been created female?" Attitudes are contagious: with our spouses, our children if we are married; with the men we meet if we are single.

How Can a Woman Look "More Feminine?" There are so many ways a woman can enhance her feminine characteristics. (And interestingly, many of them also make an older woman appear younger.) First of all, she can choose clothes in softer fabrics which fit well, emphasizing natural feminine curves without being too revealing. High heels definitely look more feminine and make a woman take shorter steps, so her walk is daintier. (A slingback is especially good.) Softer, longer, curled hairstyles also accentuate femininity.

You can relieve the severity of an "office uniform" by looking for curved lines rather than angular lines in jackets. A rounded jacket bottom or collar, for instance, is more feminine. Well-coordinated separates, as a change from the matched suit, are also younger, brighter. So, too, are short jackets or peplum jackets. And do seek a graceful fullness to a skirt.

Look for softness in a blouse. It needn't be ruffly, but the fabric can drape or tie in a fluid way.

Sometimes just a few simple adornments can help you retain your gender: a lovely silk scarf around your neck; a beautiful bracelet or necklace; a soft belt; a flash of gold or silver at your ears.

Even pants need not look "masculine," if they are well cut and perhaps relieved with pleats—if they're appropriate to your figure. It helps, too, to wear pants together with heels and frankly feminine tops and accessories.

In choosing colors, remember that unrelieved neutrals and dark shades can be mannish. Look for soft pastels as well as bright shades.

Now, here are some specific tips for the various style types.

The Feminine/Romantic is, by definition, the epitome of femininity; no problems here.

But the Town and Country or Petite Natural tends to be the most "Unisex." She can feminize herself by avoiding short and severe haircuts, though she does tend to prefer them. Sometimes a wash-and-wear body perm can give the easy care she loves, while appearing less boyish. More accessories (consider piercing the ears so earrings are easy to wear) and a touch of makeup are also helpful. And in clothes, rather than reaching for boys' pants, strive for the greater refinement, the good tweeds and plaids and nubby textures of the Town and Country look.

The Classic/Sophisticate is sometimes *so* classic and stately that she's intimidating and unapproachable as a woman. If she'll "think soft" by adding a flower, a bow, pearls, rounder lines, and softer finishes to her fabrics, she'll look much more feminine. I've seen a big change effected simply by substituting pearl button earrings for gold hoops and frameless glasses for hard frames.

The Youthful Romantic has no trouble looking feminine, but she tends to be girlish and thus may have a problem being taken seriously. Also, she may come across as prissy Victorian. Looking for more flowing, looser lines, and adding color and accessories will help her womanly image.

The Dramatic woman become less feminine only if she buys into fashion so totally that she negates her femaleness. She needs to watch out for severity, too-strong colors, and offensively long fingernails, and to avoid excessive statements in jewelry. (Save the necklace made of bones and teeth for a costume party.) What is appropriate for her in the beauty business or theatrical world may be inappropriate for a social situation. Toning it down is the key for her.

The World of Singles: Clothes Do Talk! What about clothes in the world of singles? How can you appeal to the "right" sort of man for you?

We've talked a lot about women's personality style types. Did it occur to you in reading this that men also tend to fall into distinct categories which correspond to four of the feminine types? They definitely do. And in my classes, countless men relate to this and for the first time understand why they choose specific clothing.

What's more, men and women within the same style types tend to be attracted to one another. What we project, we tend to get back.

Here's how it works.

Mr. Elegant: the Clark Gable type. This suave man, with his well-bred manner and well-tailored apparel, is frequently drawn to the Classic/Sophisticate or the Feminine/Romantic woman.

The Outdoorsman: the lumberjack, rugged outdoorsman. He's usually low-key, often wears a beard, jeans, boots, and hates a shirt and tie. He likes the Town and Country/Natural woman.

The Adventurer: the Warren Beatty or Burt Reynolds character. He may wear gold medallions, silk open-neck shirts, and shoes with heels. He's usually attracted to the Dramatic woman.

The Conservative: the IBM executive, Ivy League, button-down-collar man. This Walter Cronkite-Gerald Ford type tends to prefer the Youthful Romantic sort of woman.

So if you find you're attracting a guy whose idea of fun is taking you back-packing, and you'd much prefer a quiet, elegant dinner date, take a look at how you present yourself. Is your casual, artless dressing drawing the Outdoorsman? Is what you wear really true to who you are today?

On the other hand, if you're a soft, romantic woman in strappy sandals and soft ruffles, it's probably a waste of your time to wait for a call from the man you met last night—the one in the jeans and plaid shirt. Possibly your images are out of sync, even though he probably could not verbalize it; he knows simply by looking at you. It's the old making-up-your-mind-in-ninety-seconds principle which we discussed in chapter 1—the "packaging," the language of clothes.

It doesn't seem fair, does it? But whether we like it or not, it's the nature of man.

Moreover, if you're a single working woman, striving to get ahead, and perhaps even competing with men, you may have to decide whether you would prefer a particular man to shake your hand or to put his arm around you. It's very difficult to have it both ways at the same time: to work as an equal or to compete with men and also to expect to arouse warm, tender feelings. Possibly you'll have to count the cost of "dressing for success" in terms of appealing to men.

Suppose, however, that you are seriously dating someone, or even are already married, and you and the man you love have different ideas on how you should dress. Sometimes a man relates to you in terms of what his mother wore, or some other stereotyped idea of what women "should" wear. I've seen many women trapped by, "My husband likes/doesn't like...." But I find that when you look *terrific*—even if it's different from your man's ideas, he'll love what you wear. (I've also had husbands tell me they hate makeup, but when their wives came home from a Uniquely You makeup workshop looking wonderful, but not "made up," they liked what they saw.)

Certainly you need to dress first for the person you are; but if you dress *only* for yourself, you may be losing an opportunity to really please and uplift the man in your life. So do listen to what he likes. If, for instance, he thinks a certain dress looks "school marmish," wear it for daytime occasions when you're not together. If your ideas seem to differ a lot, learn to compromise. For example, if he says he wants you to look "sexy," see if he'll settle for a dress which drapes softly or one which is stunning and in good taste without being overtly provocative.

I've learned to soften my own classic image at home, because my husband likes a more romantic look; and he truly appreciates my making the effort.

Remember, too, if you genuinely try to please him with your wardrobe, he may be more open to your suggestions for him.

Helping Your Mate Dress Appropriately. If you're married, take a good look at the foregoing masculine style types and see which seems to best describe your husband. You might be able to help him present a believable image in business by encouraging him to dress in a way which is compatible with his basic personality.

Do be careful, however, not to come on as critical. And be sure he *wants* you to be his "helper" in this department. Some men have definite ideas and would resent your efforts. But many hate to be bothered and would welcome your assistance.

Some men think spending time on their appearance is effeminate. But as Egon Von Furstenberg points out in *The Power Look*, what actually happens is that, "Not caring reflects a fear of success, an unwillingness to compete with the top men."

Men, he notes, tend to forget that "Their clothes convey their achievements and self-respect to the world every day." They're inclined to spend money on cars, cameras, TV, sports equipment, but not on clothes.

Here are some general guidelines on clothes which are compatible with different masculine style types.

Mr. Elegant requires crisp, precise tailoring and may look well in double-breasted cuts and neat, small, clearly defined patterns.

The Adventurer loves to be noticed for his individuality, flair, and energy. He's probably already expressing these qualities in his selection of clothes. (You may want to try subtly to tone him down a little if he's in corporate business.)

The Outdoorsman, if he must wear a suit, looks best in single-breasted jackets and bolder, more rugged fabrics. Medium tones and heathery blends of color give a less urban look.

The Conservative, defined by Von Furstenberg as "a low profile expression of personal competence," should choose solid colors and understated patterns.

Now, here are some additional pointers for helping the man (or men, if you have sons!) in your life to shop wisely.

TIPS ON CHOOSING MEN'S CLOTHING

- A tall, thin, long-boned man can look broader if he wears contrasting color jacket and pants and chooses medium to light color tones and heavier textures.
- A thick body build looks taller and thinner in monochromatic colors, single-breasted suits, natural shoulders. Choose smooth or matte-finish fabrics and avoid patch pockets and pin stripes.

TO DRESS FOR SUCCESS:

- Dress as well as your client.
- Avoid double knits if you're a corporate executive or would-be executive.
- Wear only jewelry which is functional.
- Avoid feminine items.
- Don't wear green, purple, mustard. (All brought negative response in John Malloy's intensive testing, detailed in *Dress for Success*.)
- Remember that removing your jacket weakens your "authority."
- A regimental striped tie suggests good education, Ivy league.
- Choose knee-length socks so the leg doesn't show when you sit down or cross your legs.
- You'll be taken more seriously if you wear a dark suit.
- A white shirt still brings the best response for taste and credibility.

Men who look successful and well educated, says Malloy, receive preferential treatment in almost all social and business encounters.

Another important way you can assist your husband in dressing for success is to encourage and help him keep his clothes in top condition. Details do make a difference. Others notice shoes which are shined and newly heeled. (In fact, one executive told me he gets his strongest impressions about people from their shoes. "If they're shabby, even if the man wears a new suit, I figure it's his only suit.") It's important that clothes hang well and are wrinkle free, and that shirts look crisp. Everything he wears should be checked after each wearing for spots, missing buttons, anything which needs attention.

When you help the man in your life look more like the "producer-achiever" male and when you dress to express your sensitivity, your God-given femininity, you'll see the mirror effect we've mentioned before take place. As he looks better, he'll feel better about himself as a man, and begin to treat you more like a woman—especially as *you* look (and feel) more "cherishable."

Consider the woman who vacationed in the woods with her husband. During the daytime, when she wore shorts or slacks, he walked beside her or before her, letting her fend for herself. But in the cool of the evening, she'd sometimes put on a caftan or a long wool skirt. So when they walked outside together after dinner, she truly needed his help over a fallen log, a rocky outcropping. And he gallantly gave it.

With her long skirt, she had created a visual and physical contrast to her husband. And because of it, he responded to become the protective, active male, while she became the cherished, cared-for female.

BEAUTY IS DETAIL

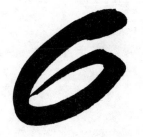

CASTING ALL YOUR CARES ON HIM

"Your hair looks just wonderful today. I like it *so* much better than the way you used to wear it."

Did anyone ever give you a message like this—in a tone which made you feel that, for years, you must have looked like a drab photo taken "before the transformation"?

Or, as you waited patiently for a car to back out of a parking space, did someone ever zoom around you and take that space?

Or have you ever worked and worked on a project—and had no one even comment on it?

Of course, those are little things. Nothing to get upset about, really. Silly even to mention.

Yet we *are* upset. Especially when these little things multiply—often to the point where we wonder if anyone really cares about us.

How fortunate we are, then, that *God does care*. He is a God of detail, and he cares about every single aspect of our being—every need, every concern. After all, he has numbered every hair of our head, we're told in Matthew 10:30. And in Psalm 56:8, we see that he is so compassionate, he doesn't overlook a single tear, but would put our "tears in a bottle."

If it matters to us, it matters to God—and that includes hair and parking places, not just life and death matters, not just momentous decisions.

Indeed, in Philippians 4:6, Paul urges us not to be anxious about anything, but "in everything by prayer and petition, with thanksgiving, present your requests to God."

Everything.

Perhaps that's because God, in his wisdom, knows how our little concerns can grow if we try to ignore them.

I learned this when I first confronted the intricacies of putting on a seminar. It's almost as complicated as planning a wedding, and things do go wrong. Test-lights for color profiles can burn out at the wrong time. Sometimes the hotel mixes up our reservations. An irate person disrupts the continuity. I never know what will happen. No two are the same.

I remember one day-long seminar at which I expected VIPs to attend. I arrived tired; one of my consultants called in sick at the last minute; I realized someone had borrowed the color testers. And to top it all off, there was a mouse in the room.

With ten minutes to go, I was in tears and praying, "How, Lord, am I going to pull this together?"

Not a moment later, a consultant I hadn't expected arrived, and she had testers in her car.

Truly, God does handle problems which are beyond our control. And there is nothing like the peace of knowing that he takes care of it all—every tiny detail.

God deeply desires that we not let our worries get out of hand but that we take them all to him and communicate exactly how we feel. David urged that we trust him at all times and "pour out your hearts to him, for God is our refuge" (Psalm 62:8).

Moreover, because no one knows us better than God (the Psalmist says all our ways are known to him) we can take the innermost thoughts of our beings to him. We can share those hidden yearnings and fears and cares which perhaps we can't express to anyone else.

What a wonderfully aware and totally concerned God we have, that we may be invited to cast all (yes, it says *all*) our anxieties on him, for he cares for us! (1 Peter 5:7).

And just as he knows how little concerns can escalate, he knows how those little transgressions can grow and contaminate our inner beauty.

Solomon understood this when he stated in Ecclesiastes 10:1 that "A little folly outweighs wisdom and honor."

It's important, then, that just as we cast our cares on him, we also cast all our follies to God. For he is not a "gotcha" God, but "faithful and just and will forgive us" (1 John 1:9).

We can repeat David's plea of Psalm 139:23, 24: "Search me, O God, and know my heart; test me and know my anxious thoughts. See if there is any offensive way in me."

He'll help us see those well-hidden problem areas, so that we can present them and be free of them.

What an amazing God! He cares about every detail, and he *takes* care of every detail of our lives!

If you don't have a sense of his closeness in your life, I want to encourage you to reach out to him with the details which concern you—to ask for his presence in your life.

ABOUT "ADORNMENTS"

A gold chain to fill in a neckline ... a little mascara to accent the eyes ... a soft hairstyle to relieve an angular face. It's those external details which polish our "look."

And most of us love these extra touches. Our womanly desire for adornment is, in fact, deeply rooted in the biblical past. In Genesis, Abraham's servant, seeking a wife for Isaac, brought out gold and silver jewelry and clothing for Rebekah. In Exodus, God told Moses that when his people left Egypt, they should not go empty-handed, but every woman would ask for jewels, silver, gold, and clothing from the Egyptians. Isaiah mentions how "a bride adorns herself with her jewels."

Moreover, in the "Song of Songs," Solomon declares to his beloved, "Your cheeks are beautiful with earrings, your neck with strings of jewels. We will make you earrings of gold, studded with silver."

However, in the New Testament, both 1 Peter 3:3, 4 and 1 Timothy 2:9 caution women about wearing braided hair and gold. In 1 Timothy Paul urges that they adorn themselves with *modesty*, which my dictionary defines as "restraint; free from anything suggestive of sexual impurity."

Indeed, according to Paul Brand and Philip Yancey, writing in *Fearfully and Wonderfully Made*, in Paul's time, women who dressed their hair in a certain manner might be assumed to be sexually impure; they were usually either prostitutes or pagan priestesses.

Today hairstyle and gold jewelry certainly don't identify us in such a manner. Even so, we'd be wise to concern ourselves with adorning our persons with "modesty" in the sense of restraint. The Bible again and again points us toward moderation in all things. And we've all seen the gaudiness of the woman decked out like the proverbial Christmas tree.

So first, look at yourself objectively. You know more than you may think you do. Then, resist the temptation to add more and more (earrings, necklace, bracelets, rings, scarf, belt, bows, pins). Remember that less is more, and that there is elegance in restraint.

Accessories. When you select accessories—that is, everything above and beyond your basic outfit of suit and blouse, or dress—when does "more" become too much?

A simple way to establish a guideline is actually to tally or count all the details.

Here is a suggested guide to help you see if you ever tend to become carried away.

ACCESSORY GUIDE
Score one point for each of the following:

Every color in your total costume
Each plain, simple shoe
Any arresting detail on your shoes (bows, buckles, multi-colors, open toes, open heels, chains, rope)
Stockings *if* they are colored, patterned, or jeweled, rather than skin tone
Buttons, if a different color than garment
Jewelry (watches, bracelets, chains, earrings, pins)
Bows, ruffles, contrasting belts
Glasses (add another point if they are unusual, eye-catching)
Hat
Handbag (add extra points if it has bright hardware, chains, buckles, extra colors)
Bright red hair
Bright-colored fingernails
Bright-colored toenails (if they show)

If your total count is 11 to 13, you will not be over-accessorized. If it's under eight, you're probably understated, possibly a tad boring. If it's higher, think about what you might eliminate. You can be simply beautiful, and beautifully simple!

Just how do you select appropriate accessories? Think *style type;* think *mood;* think *proportion.*

Style type. When you accessorize an outfit, if you first consider your style type, you will choose items which are compatible with who you are and which, altogether, add to your credibility.

Remember, these suggestions are not an attempt to restrict or box you in, but to help you find accessories which agree with and complement the person you are, and which will make you more believable to others.

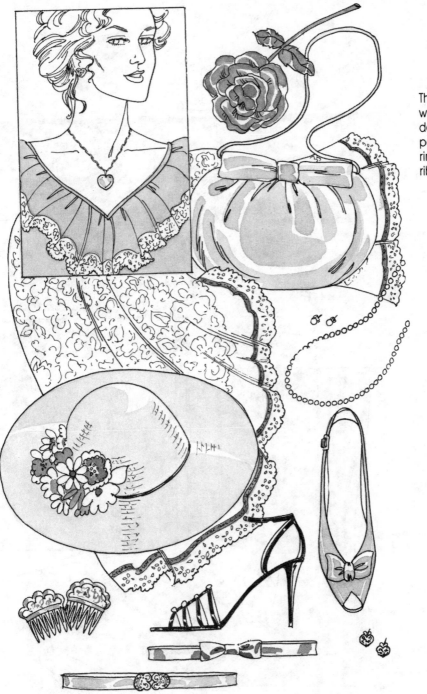

The Feminine/Romantic will select soft scarves, dainty strapped shoes, pearls, delicate earrings, silk flowers, and ribbons.

The Classic/Sophisticate will feel most comfortable in a simple, classic hat, button earrings, gold jewelry; shoes, purse, and belt which are simple but feminine.

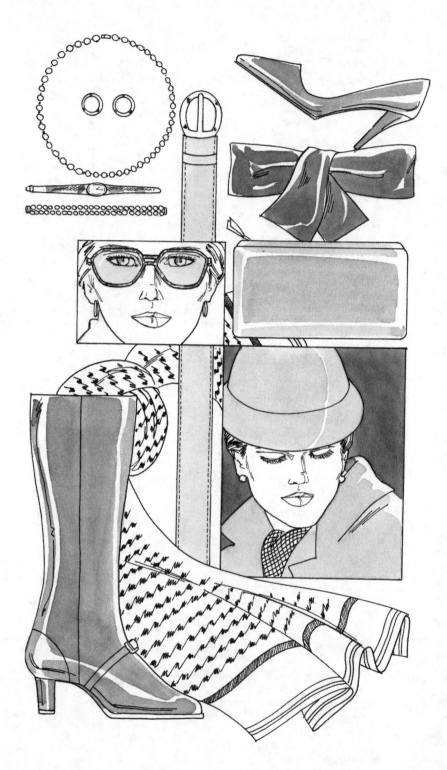

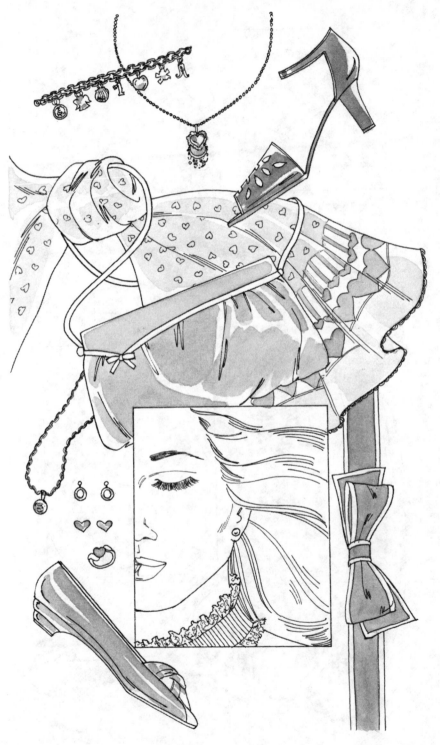

The Youthful Romantic will prefer simple button earrings, dainty chains, bows, understated shoes and purses.

The Dramatic will reach for bold jewelry, bangles—splashy, costumey, ethnic effects.

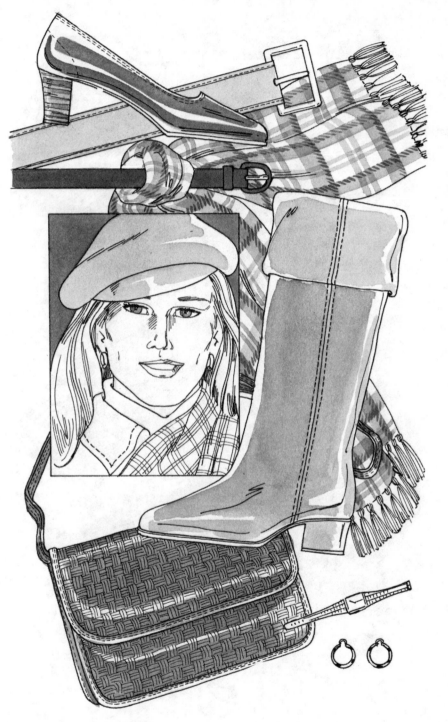

The Town and Coun-
try/Natural will seek
berets, hoop earrings,
handmade jewelry,
mostly lower-heeled
shoes and boots.

The Petite Natural, a mini version of the Town and Country/Natural, likes casual, natural accessories, understated elegance.

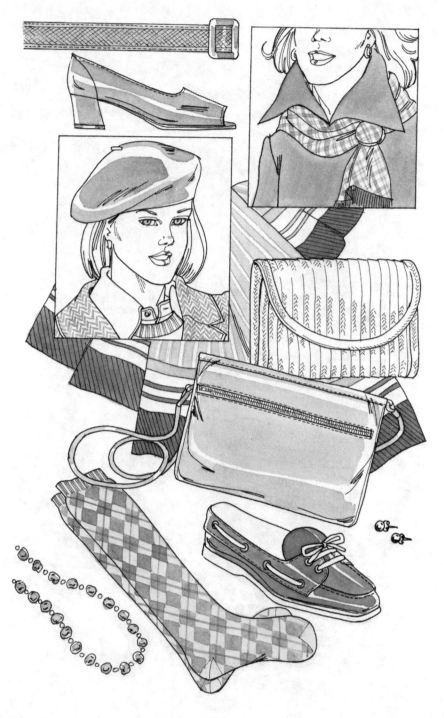

Perhaps you've wondered why certain accessories remain in your drawers. For instance, maybe you own a very modern handmade silver bracelet which you never wear. But if you're a Youthful Romantic, of course you wouldn't feel comfortable in it; it's meant for a Dramatic, or perhaps a Town and Country/Natural. Or you might be like Alice, one of our consultants in Washington, D.C., who brought in an antique pin she wanted to use. It was lovely, but it was also ridiculous on her rough-textured suit lapel. The pin, you see, was very romantic, and she is a Town and Country/Natural. She decided to take the pin home and frame it (I love to use wonderful old pins around the house in decorating—on pillows, for instance), and to buy a tailored lapel pin to wear.

Joyce, on the other hand, was true to her Dramatic style type, but like many Dramatics, she tended to overdo. The first time I saw her, she had pins, jewels, and necklaces everywhere. She must have registered twenty-five on our accessory point scale. Toned down, she is still Dramatic, but no longer makes such an overwhelming statement.

By the way, we all tend to be collectors of accessories, to have more than we can appropriately use. Like the pins, many of these can be put to use around your home. For instance, if you have a drawer full of gift scarves, fill a clear urn with them and enjoy the colors. I even made a fur piece into pillows, and they were handsome—until the dog challenged them. (The pillows lost!)

Mood. All of your accessories should be in keeping with the mood of your outfit. Is it strictly business, partygoing, or relaxed and casual?

Since shoes seem to be the most troublesome area, here's where we begin. Often we tend to put the wrong shoe with our outfits: strappy sandals with a tweed suit, for instance, or a broad-heeled pump with a dressy dress. If we compound the error with purse, jewelry, and belt in still different moods—look what a picture of confusion we present!

Be sure there's a compatibility about the details of what you wear.

For business wear, the classic pump is probably the safest style, if you can afford only one pair of shoes right now. (Avoid spike heels, clunky wooden soles, many cross-straps, vinyl, or plastic.)

Look too for shoes which do not cause the observer to see you "feet first." The key lies in wearing a shoe color which either matches the hem of your outfit or is darker. White-white calls at-

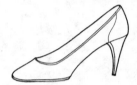

The classic pump

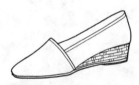

Walking shoe

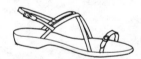

Summer sandal

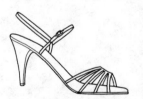

Dressy open strap

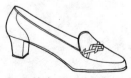

Casual shoe

tention to your feet. Try bone, beige, or taupe instead.

And by the way, a purse the same color as the shoe or lighter (but never darker) adds harmony to your total look.

Jewelry, too, should suit the mood of your outfit. Don't be like the teenager I saw recently, wearing pearls with jeans! Costume jewelry (made of wood, beads, imitation gems, nonprecious metals) is compatible with the sportive look of a blazer and skirt or slacks. However, an elegant dress or a suit of fine fabric should be complemented with fine jewelry (of precious metals such as gold, platinum, and sterling silver; precious or semiprecious gemstones, pearls).

Brushed metal is the dressiest of all, especially if it's combined with stones or pearls, while shiny metal is more appropriate for sport or casual wear. If you combine shiny and brushed metal, the look will not be as dressy.

Be sure, too, that the texture and weight of your jewelry is compatible with the texture and weight of the fabric you are wearing.

And don't worry about "matching" all your jewelry; two or three pieces of matched jewelry is plenty. Unmatched pieces can be chic, if you combine them carefully. Experiment with several necklaces or bracelets or rings worn together.

You'll find you can even create the look of "fineness" without spending thousands, if you carefully mix one or two fine pieces with good costume jewelry. For instance, you can successfully mix fourteen karat gold with well-done gold electroplate.

And by the way, if you find that you have some nice jewelry which is not appropriate to your color palette (remember, gold is best for spring and fall; silver for summer and winter), don't get rid of it. Mix your gold and silver. They'll neutralize each other, and can be very attractive together.

Scarves can be effective additions to many outfits, but be sure the texture and pattern coordinate with the dress or suit. For instance, if you wear a herringbone suit, choose a medium-weight material for the scarf (not a very light silk), and a small print which will not fight the herringbone. Also, a very soft floral print would not be appropriate with a crisply tailored suit, but a smart stripe or geometric print would be perfect. It's really a matter of common sense. Don't be like one client of mine who wore a delicate summer scarf over a heavy winter coat (or the many people I see who try to combine summer shoes with winter outfits).

Belts, too, come in so many different shapes and forms, you can add new life to an old dress if you choose carefully from the many materials. Ribbon or a fine suede, for instance, would be appropriate to a silk dress, while webbing, string, raffia, or metal links would work well with denims. Use belts to brighten your wardrobe and your life. They're fine fashion investments.

Proportion. Accessories play a far more important role in balancing your total "look," in giving you credibility, than most people realize. They also affect the overall line and shape you present to the eye.

Here are some tips for choosing shoes: You can minimize ankles and slenderize calves if you avoid high cuts and ankle straps but pick pointed toes. Eliminate shiny materials or shoes which call attention to your feet, and look for suedes or other soft finishes. Choose colors which match your outfit. Your feet will also appear slimmer if your shoes are pointed at the toe, are all one color, and have a simple, low cut.

You can broaden too-thin ankles and calves by choosing shoes with ankle straps and rounded or square toes. Select two-toned shoes in suede or soft finishes, and look for buckles and bows for width.

Also, although short women tend to wear higher heels and tall women wear lower heels—when you consider the visual effect, the reverse ought to be true. The taller you are, the higher the heels you can wear effectively. Very high heels on a tiny woman give a walking-on-stilts look. Again, it's a matter of proportion.

As for jewelry, in selecting necklaces, remember that short chains or strands of beads tend to shorten a neck (but they also tend to emphasize a double chin).

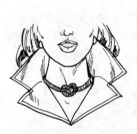

Greater length elongates and draws attention away from chin and neck. A small chain also makes the shoulders appear broader, while graduated beads are not good for narrow shoulders or a full bust, because they draw the eye to their center, and then down.

Think proportion, too, when selecting eyeglass frames. They should be as wide as the widest part of your face, and in proportion to the shape and size of your face. Follow the contour of your eyes and brows and select a high or rounded bridge for a small nose, a lower or straight bridge for a long nose. Remember, too, to blend the frame color with your complexion and your hair coloring; or, if you choose metal frames, select the metal of your season. When you shop, it's a good idea to take someone objective along to help you decide.

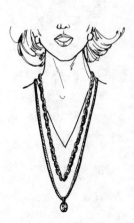

Try always to keep your accessories in scale. Delicate hoop ear-

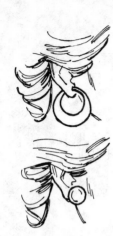

rings are fine for a petite woman, but a larger woman needs more massive earrings.

Button earrings can be proportioned to your size. These are just right for a small-to-medium-sized woman.

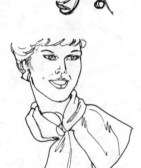

These delicate earrings demand both a petite build and delicate facial features.

Also, a bulky purse overwhelms a small stature, but is totally appropriate for a larger person.

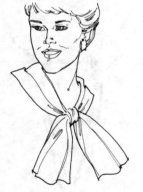

And when you wear a scarf, keep it in proportion to your upper body, as well as to the shape and size of your head. You can also use a scarf, tied high at the neckline, to cut the length of an overly long neck; or, if the scarf is long and narrow, to elongate the face and neck.

If you enjoy stoles (which can be perfect when a coat isn't appropriate but some warmth is needed), practice draping them before making a public appearance. They, too, can be used to widen or elongate.

Hats are chic and fun. They make a fashion statement by framing the face, and can make your costume more complete. But be sure the brim is not wider than your shoulders and that the crown is as wide as the widest part of your face.

Long neck

The width of your belt also affects your overall proportions. Notice how a very narrow belt makes your hips look larger, while a medium width makes them appear smaller. A wide belt, on the other hand, may make you appear short-waisted, even if you're not.

If you're large waisted, you needn't give up the fun of belts. Choose one with a handsome buckle which draws the eye and cover your sides with an open sweater, vest, or jacket.

I know I've given you what may seem an enormous number of things to think about in working out the details of your appearance.

To summarize and help you with your shopping, here are the main points to keep in mind when looking for accessories.

Short neck

1. Use your style type as a guide when you buy.
2. Consider the mood of the outfit(s) you're accessorizing.
3. Remember your body size and shape: use accessories in order to flatter it.
4. Look for items which harmonize with each other and can be worn with more than one costume.
5. Remember your best colors and stick to them.
6. Look for lasting value and quality.
7. Keep the center of interest in one area at a time. (Don't wear

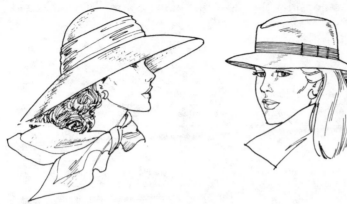

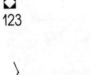

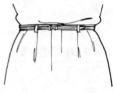

an eye-catching belt *and* an elaborate necklace.)

8. Repeat an accessory color only three times, unless you want a patchwork quilt effect.
9. Any color in an accessory should be repeated and balanced (using a similar quantity) once more in your outfit.
10. Remember that fine quality accessories with clean lines can make inexpensive clothes look better . . .

. . . while extremes in shape and detailing, tacky materials can spoil the effect of even the finest of clothes.

MAKEUP

Do you know that makeup is "biblical"?

Well, in the Book of 2 Samuel, Joab sent the wise woman to the king, cautioning her to "pretend you're in mourning and don't use any cosmetic lotions."

Obviously, "cosmetic lotions" were the norm at the time. But not so long ago, it seemed that many Christian women looked as though *they* were in mourning. Indeed, the image of a "Christian woman" was a colorless female with her hair pulled back into a tight bun.

That's no longer true in most churches, and a number of pastors can be heard declaring that "a little paint on the barn" is, indeed, desirable.

Makeup, correctly applied, will not make you look "made up." Instead, it will enhance the unique coloring, the unique features you have, accenting the positive, minimizing the not-so-positive. Did you know that the root word of "cosmetics" is the Greek word *kosmos*, meaning order, harmony? *Cosmetics* thus can bring order out of chaos!

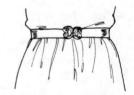

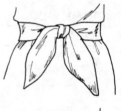

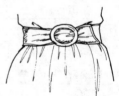

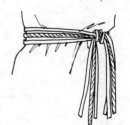

First, let's consider the most becoming colors for your season.

COSMETIC PROFILE

AUTUMN EYESHADOW

EYE COLOR	Brown	Amber	Green	Blue
UNDER BROW	Beige	Beige	Beige	Beige
ORBITAL BONE	Bronze Rum raisin	Bronze	Cedar	Cedar
LID	Smoky green Khaki smoke Smoky amethyst	Fern green Khaki smoke Bronze	Fern green Smoky green	Adriatic Deep sea
LINER	Sable	Brown frost	Olive	Dark teal

SPRING EYESHADOW

EYE COLOR	Brown	Amber	Blue	Green
UNDER BROW	Beige	Beige	Beige	Beige
ORBITAL BONE	Cedar	Cedar	Dawn	Cedar
LID	Antique violet Khaki smoke	Violet Fern green	Dresden blue	Fern green
LINER	Brown frost Taupe		Teal Slate	Avocado Taupe

WINTER EYESHADOW

EYE COLOR	Brown	Brown/green	Gray/blue	Gray/green
UNDER BROW	Beige	Beige	Diamond	Beige
ORBITAL BONE	Rum raisin	Rum raisin	Gray	Gray, dawn
LID	Khaki smoke Smoky amethyst	Smoky green Smoky amethyst	Dresden blue Gray, wedgewood	Fern green Smoky green
LINER	Sable, black Plum brown	Charcoal frost	Smoke	Avocado

SUMMER EYESHADOW

EYE COLOR	Blue Gray/blue	Aqua/blue	Green	Brown
UNDER BROW	Beige	Beige	Beige	Beige
ORBITAL BONE	Dawn	Dawn	Dawn	Dawn
LID	Dresden blue Wedgewood	Deep sea Wedgewood	Fern green Khaki smoke	Smoky amethyst Smoky green
LINER	Teal	Dark teal Teal	Avocado	Antique violet Brown plum

	LIPSTICK	**BLUSHER**
AUTUMN	shades of orange, or: mocha, rust, brown no blue tones	dark peach or russet, salmon, soft red no blue tones
SPRING	light peach, coral, or coral pink no blue tones	peach, light rust, salmon no blue tones
WINTER	shades of pink or true red no orange tones	shades of red no orange tones
SUMMER	light to medium pink, burgundy, blue red, plum no orange tones	pink or plum, burgundy, blue red no orange tones

Now, how do you apply that color? Let's think first about what you're working with and take an honest look at your facial shape and features.

What is the basic shape of your face? There are seven basic shapes, one of which most closely resembles yours. Pull your hair back and take a good look to see which of these illustrations on the next page comes closest to your shape. If you're in doubt, trace the outline of your face on the mirror with soap.

Now that you have determined what the shape of your face is, begin with:

Foundation color, to give your face a smooth, even look and to hide imperfections. Select the closest color to your natural skin. Avoid the trap of using a darker shade to achieve "more color." Instead, you'll add color with a light application of blusher or rouge.

Place dots of foundation on your chin, cheeks, nose, and forehead. Avoid rubbing it in. Blend evenly with upward strokes. Think of it as icing a cake! Use your ring finger to smooth around the eyes. Do *not* use foundation on your neck, but blend carefully at the jawbone.

Rouge or blusher will add sparkle to your eyes, youthful color to your face. Be sure the color is compatible with your natural skin tones.

Now, place it correctly on the cheekbone. If you apply below the cheekbone, you'll create a sagging line. Apply your blusher on the rounded area which is defined when you smile. In general, and particularly if your face is oval, start directly below the iris of your eye and blend all the way to the hairline and to within a finger's width of the eye.

OVAL: The "ideal" face shape. Forehead is wider than chin, cheekbones dominant, and face gracefully tapers from cheeks to a narrower oval chin.

RECTANGULAR: This face is long and squared. Forehead is approximately the same width as cheekbones and jawline.

SQUARE: The squared forehead is about the same width as the cheekbones and jawline. A strong, square jaw is the dominant feature.

ROUND: The round face is almost as wide as it is long, with greatest width at the cheeks.

HEART/TRIANGLE: This face shape has a wide forehead and high cheekbones, and tapers down to a narrow chin.

DIAMOND: Similar to the oval, this face differs because the cheeks are considerably wider. They taper both to the forehead and the chin.

PEAR: Notable for its broad jawline and narrow forehead, this face shape is the inverse of the heart/triangle.

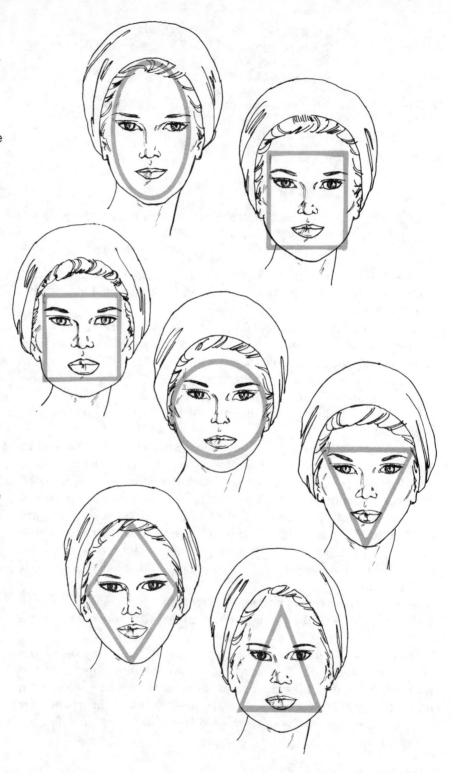

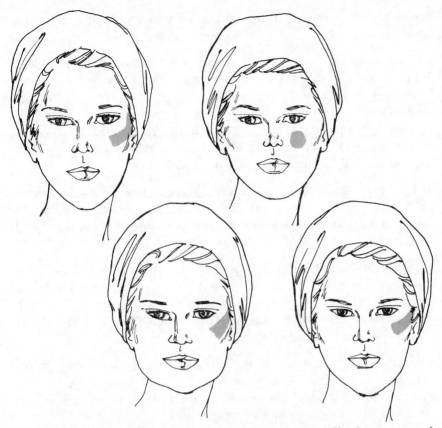

If your face is *long*, begin your blusher just behind the fleshy portion of the cheek which shows when you smile. Extend it up to the temple, as shown.

If your face is *round*, apply blusher directly on the rounded cheek area which is obvious when you smile. Do not extend it to the hairline. Keep the color at the center of the face.

If your face is *square*, begin your blusher at the top of the round of the cheek. Follow the highest portion of the cheekbone, blending the blusher almost, but not all the way, to the temple.

And here is your guide for an *oval*-shaped face.

Whatever your face shape, always blend carefully for a natural look, without a harsh "slash" or circle of color effect. Use a second mirror to check yourself in profile to be sure.

Eye makeup will accent the color of your eyes and open them as the "window of your being."

Rather than coordinating your eye shadow with the color of your outfit, choose a color which most closely matches your eyes. It will intensify their color and be correct with all of your wardrobe. Frosted shadow reflects light and tends to show lines, so wear it only if you have no lines to reveal. Apply the shadow on the lid directly above the eye. Then, if you wish to further accent your eyes, apply a neutral shadow to soften, just above the lid. You may also use a light highlight just under the brow to lift a droopy lid.

Here are some other ways to enhance eyes of different shapes and contexts.

If your eyes have *droopy lids:* Make a pencil line just above the upper lashes. But instead of penciling to the outer edge of the lid

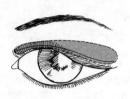

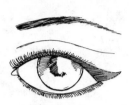

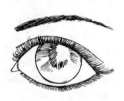

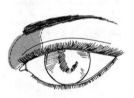

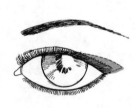

where the eye droops, lift up the corner: pencil up and out. Do not apply shadow or mascara to the outer corner.

If your eyes are *deep-set:* Use a light shadow on the entire upper lid and on your brow bone. Apply your pencil close to your upper lashes, extending the line up and out at the outer corner of the eye. You will actually create a triangle of color between the outer corner of your eye, a point directly above it in the crease, and the top edge of the last lash. Fill this in with shadow and blend carefully. Use mascara mainly on tips of top and lower lashes.

If your eyes are *round:* Use a pencil directly next to the lashes on the upper lid. Place a dot at the edge of the eye where your last lash touches your brow bone. Extend your liner to this point and blend it. Use a pencil under lower lashes.

If your eyes are *oriental:* Use a medium eye shadow on the inner corner. (This helps define the nose.) Apply a light-toned shadow over the entire lid. To create an eyelid "crease," draw a pencil line at the base of the brow bone. Apply liner close to upper and lower lashes. Mascara all lashes lightly.

If your eyes are *almond shaped:* Use a deeper-toned shadow on the outer portion of the lid and extend it a little. A light-toned shadow on the inner corner should extend to the brow bone. Apply mascara to both upper and lower lashes.

Eyebrow pencil defines and accents the brow. Apply it in short strokes in the same direction that brow hairs grow. Then brush your brows to blend in.

If your brows are very sparse, use two shades of eyebrow pencil: one to match your hair, and one which is lighter.

You may also want to shape your brows by plucking. But whether you pluck to eliminate or pencil-in to thicken, be sure to keep the size of your brows proportionate to your face. Petite features, for instance, can be overwhelmed by bushy brows.

In shaping your brows, start directly over the inner end of the eye. This will be the thickest part of your brow. Arch it so the highest point is in line with the outer edge of your iris—the colored part of your eye. Curve the brow out and slightly down, ending at a point which you can determine by holding a pencil or drawing an imaginary line from your nostril to the outer corner of your eye.

As for mascara, which makes your lashes look thicker, fuller, longer, choose a color which matches your lashes unless they are very pale, in which case, go for medium brown. Black at the tip of brown lashes will make them look longer. Also, you might enjoy trying a mascara in a blue or green tone. Surprisingly, it won't look "colored," and it will enhance your eye color.

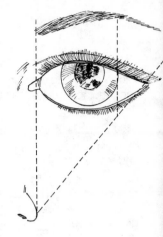

Lipstick gives your lips soft, smooth, moist color and sheen and will also protect them from chapping. A lip-liner pencil is useful not only for defining the contours of the lip; it also keeps your lipstick from bleeding above or below the lipline.

You can also change the shape of your lips by using a neutral lipliner pencil. If, for instance, you feel your lips are too full, line just inside the edge with the pencil and fill in with the lipstick. If you think they're too thin, use the liner just outside the edge of the lip. And if your lips are not quite symmetrical, line both sides to match and fill in with lipstick. If your lips are fuller at the top or bottom, you can either enlarge the thinner part, or thin the fuller to make the total lip better balanced.

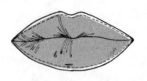

Are you hesitant to try this? Many women are, but it really works and doesn't look artificial.

Shading cream is a soft, putty-like cream which can effectively conceal, cover, and sculpt. Some women enjoy using it to contour their faces for special occasions. Two basic principles to remember: light shading cream brings features forward, while darker cream pushes them back.

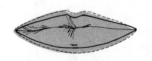

Using the highlighting cream, many women are pleased to find that they can minimize the "laugh lines" which extend down from the nose on either side of the mouth, as well as reduce any indentation above the chin.

Highlighter can also de-emphasize a low bridge on the nose, circles under the eyes, crow's feet, and forehead lines. If you use contouring highlighter at the top of your hairline, it will heighten your forehead. At the sides, it will make your forehead appear wider. And on the sides of the face, it also adds width. Highlighter will bring forward a deep-set eye, and it will even "lift up" the cheek bone if it's applied along the bone. (Use your blusher under the highlighter.)

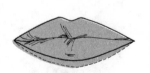

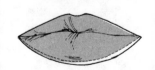

Dark shading cream, carefully blended at the side of the jaw, can help you to soften a square jaw. Beneath the chin, it can minimize a double chin. On the brow bone, it pushes back a protruding brow. Applied to the sides of the face, it thins the face; and if you use it at the very top of your forehead, it will lower a high forehead. To shorten your nose, apply the dark shading cream at the tip of the

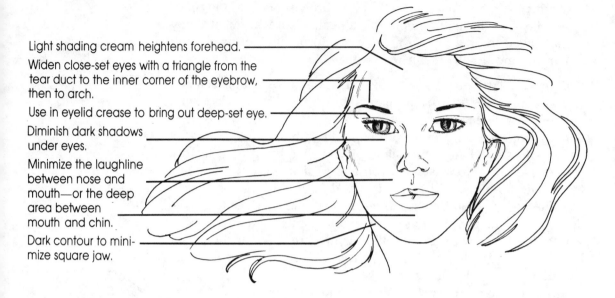

Light shading cream heightens forehead.

Widen close-set eyes with a triangle from the tear duct to the inner corner of the eyebrow, then to arch.

Use in eyelid crease to bring out deep-set eye.

Diminish dark shadows under eyes.

Minimize the laughline between nose and mouth—or the deep area between mouth and chin.

Dark contour to minimize square jaw.

nose. And to straighten a crooked nose, darken one side in the direction it's bent and lighten the opposite side.

When you apply your makeup, do be sure you work in a good light. If it's daytime, double-check yourself in the daylight before you go out.

If you wear glasses, by all means use a magnifying mirror, or buy yourself those special makeup glasses with the lenses that flip up and down.

Check yourself, too, in profile, by using a hand mirror or a three-way mirror. Other people don't just see you face-to-face, you know.

It's so exciting to see the difference the proper makeup, skillfully applied, can make in a woman's appearance. Many find that even men who insist that they hate makeup will love the way their wives look, because they're not "painted," but glowing in a natural way.

It's a pleasure to work with a woman like Judy, who at first overdid her makeup. Now all the cheapness is gone, and she has a soft, peaches and cream look which is so much more appealing.

I've seen women with rough-textured skin become much smoother in appearance once we gave them a foundation which truly blends with their skin color. We've taught a very attractive woman whose face was marred only by a crooked nose (she broke it playing volleyball) to use shading cream to "straighten" that nose. And Marian, who had a cleft chin which she felt looked too masculine, also learned to minimize it with shading cream.

We've assisted women in minimizing any tendency to a sickly sallowness with the right shades of foundation, blusher, and lipstick. And we've shown women who looked perpetually unhappy how to do away with their frowny countenance by carefully plucking their heavy brows.

HAIR

Hair Styling. Your key to a hairstyle is not what your friend wears or the latest cut advertised by a famous-name salon. It's your style type (which we've discussed earlier), and even more important, your face shape.

If your face is *oval,* you can wear many different styles, including such extremes as the dramatic drawn-straight-back look (if your features are even and well proportioned). If you feel your features are less than perfect, you'll do better with softer styles.

If your face is *oblong* or *rectangular,* try to minimize its length and accent its width. With minimum height at the top, work for fullness at the sides. Part your hair on the side, or wear bangs. Avoid a center part and long hair, unless you keep the hair around the face shorter and fuller.

If your face is *square,* work toward additional height and avoid fullness at the jaw line. Assymmetrical lines are best, and be sure not to bare the entire forehead hairline or to wear a very low part.

If your face is *round,* do everything you can to elongate. Add height at the crown and keep any fullness above the ears. Dip or wave your hair onto the cheeks to thin your face, and don't pull the hair entirely away from the face. A side part should angle up toward the crown, and a center part will be effective only if your hair covers the sides of the forehead and face.

If your face is a *triangle* or *pear,* cover the broad base with hair which lies partly over the ears and close to the cheek line. Broaden the top with curled or wispy bangs which flare toward each side.

If your face is a *heart* or *inverted triangle,* the opposite will be true. Long, loose hair adds width at the jaw line, but you'll want to avoid low parts or any curls or bangs which give a top-heavy look.

If your face is a *diamond,* work toward broadening both the jaw and forehead so they balance with the cheek. Strive for symmetrical lines. Add width at the forehead with soft, swirled bangs and by keeping hair full at the temples. Partially cover the cheeks and add fullness at the jawline.

As we've seen in chapter 4, God doesn't goof. He knows how to perfectly combine the colors of our hair, skin, and eyes. I've yet to meet a person whose natural hair color was not beautifully in harmony with the color of his or her eyes and skin.

But when we begin coloring our hair, thinking we might improve on what he gave us—woe! The results can be a disaster.

Let me be clear: I am not in any way opposed to dyeing or tinting the hair, but I am very concerned about trying to effect drastic changes.

The key to success is not to deviate sharply from your natural color. It's particularly important to stick to the same undertone, so your hair will remain compatible with your eyes and skin.

Many women have given us difficulty with their color palette because they've changed ash blonde hair to golden blonde, dark ash brown to auburn, or graying brown to black.

So if you're a winter or summer, try not to stray from the cool tones, and avoid a red henna. On the other hand, henna may be appropriate for autumns; and both springs and autumns will find warm, golden tones most becoming.

If you're a mature woman you'll look best in colors which are just a touch lighter than your original color. Darker shades can age the face.

I'm glad to see there's a growing trend toward considering gray as gorgeous, and it truly can be. One of my clients, who had to wear wigs, came to me in an ash brown wig, which, though it was the original tone of her hair, was now too harsh. We switched her to gray, and she actually looked ten years younger. You see, nature prepares your skin to be compatible with the graying of your hair.

This means that if you "hate that gray" and want to color your hair, you must be careful to choose a color which is soft and not harsh around your skin—neither too bright nor too dark.

If you look at the natural color of your hair, you'll see that it is actually a combination of several different colors—as many as five or seven. This is why it's important to seek a professional hair colorist who will use several colors of dye for a most natural look.

Do you feel a bit overwhelmed? We've packed a lot of material into this section, and it will not all come together for you immediately. Work at it as you'd eat an elephant: a little bit at a time.

BEAUTY IS ELIMINATING

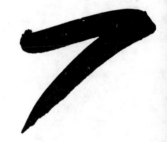

GETTING RID OF THE OLD DATA

A woman just home from an "outward bound" wilderness experience told of her first attempt at mountain climbing.

"I was fine if I concentrated on what I was doing and looked ahead. But if I looked back, it was a disaster."

Later, she saw a distinct parallel between this adventure and her own life. "I can't spend my time looking back. I have to concentrate on now—and what's ahead."

Isn't that true for all of us? Yet we tend to weigh ourselves down with what we were yesterday, protecting ourselves with the familiar and well-worn armor of past thoughts and emotions.

If we insist upon overloading ourselves with what we were, how will we be able to be what we are—or what we can become?

In 2 Corinthians 5:17 we are promised: "If anyone is in Christ, he is a new creation; the old has gone, the new has come!"

In other words, when you believe in Christ you are a new person.

Isn't it time, then, for us to *allow* the old to pass away? Let's bring what psychologists call "the old tapes" (lingering angers and hurts, destructive thought patterns) out of our inner closet, just as we do when we clean our clothes closet.

What sort of old things?

Crushing statements others have made which echo and reecho in our minds: "Don't be so stupid. Can't you ever do anything right?" "Stop being such a fool." "You've made it impossible for me to realize any of my ambitions." "I wish you were dead!"

Our own "failures": the time we were so upset we wept, or so angry we shouted during a board meeting; terrible things *we* said or did which haunt us.

Devastating disappointments: the job or recognition we didn't get and which we really deserved; that great, great love to whom we gave everything, only to have him walk away.

Profound losses, as we grieve and grieve and *grieve* for that baby which might have been; that beloved one plucked from us in sudden, much-too-early death.

And so much more. . . .

Again and again, I see women who want help in cleaning out their clothes closets so they can start over. But what they really need is to start with their inner closets.

To begin your own inner closet cleaning, ask yourself what upsets you repeatedly, what you worry about again and again, what troubled dreams you dream, what irrational fears you may have. Perhaps reading a book, such as *Discovering Yourself: The Key to Understanding Others* (Bob Rigdon, Tyndale House Publishers, 1982) will help you pinpoint trouble areas.

Also, ask trusted friends what patterns they observe which bring you repeated unhappiness. Do you, for instance, fear failure so much that it inevitably comes? Do jealousies drive you to demand attention and be possessive of friends or family members? Do old angers surface again and again?

And certainly ask the Lord to reveal to you old hurts which you may have thrust back into the darker corners of your "closet."

Now, armed with the love of the Lord—the perfect love which casts out fear—look at these painful areas just as you look at clothes which you bring out of your closet. Give them your most critical eye.

Ask yourself:

Do they fit the "new person" I am as a believer today?

Do they enhance my inner beauty?

Do I feel wonderful when I "wear" them?

If not, do what you do with ill-fitting, color-me-ugly clothes. *Give them away!*

Do you know that in the word, "forgive," the prefix "for" means "away"? So to forgive is to give away, to give up. It means to be rid of, liberated from, released from, no longer enslaved by.

So forgiveness is essential. First, let's forgive *ourselves* for the hurtful words which never can be retracted . . . the pain we've caused others . . . the things we wish we'd done—or not done.

And let's ask God to make us willing to forgive others. It's not only freeing to us. (Whom do we hurt when we fail to forgive?

Ourselves!) For he's told us to be forgiving of one another, "even as Christ has forgiven you" (Ephesians 4:32).

Another way we can give our hurts away is to release our *pride* to God. For if we're honest, often our greatest distress stems from wounded pride. ("And I thought he really loved me!" Or, "How can I ever face those people again?")

Solomon warned us a number of times in Proverbs of the problems of pride. And in the New Testament, we learn that if we humble ourselves in the sight of the Lord, he will lift us up (James 4:10). So in a sense, the way to up is, first, down. God promises to give strength to the humble (James 4:6).

And finally, we can give away our old destructive behavior patterns by presenting them as a *sacrifice*.

Why a sacrifice? Because often, we hug these old hurts to ourselves, playing and replaying the record, wearing the groove deeper and deeper. The sound of them becomes so familiar that there is a distorted comfort in their discomfort—so much so that we don't really *want* to let them go.

For instance, for a long time—before I realized it was OK to have a happy marriage, a wonderful child, to be successful—I was "happiest" in stress and panic. It was, in a sense, my comfort zone, because I was unwilling to stretch out and grow.

Muriel Cook expressed this well in a seminar on "Kitchen Table Counseling," emphasizing how we frequently "try" to give old wounds up—and then snatch them back.

But to give them to him as a gift, an offering because *he* wants them (even though they're not a "good gift" in our eyes)—ah, that is different. Once they are freely and truly sacrificed, shouldn't and wouldn't we be ashamed to take them back?

In Isaiah 43:18, 19, we are urged to "remember not the former things, nor consider the things of old. Behold, I am doing a new thing; now it springs forth, do you not perceive it? I will make a way in the wilderness and rivers in the desert" (RSV).

When we give away those malignant, destructive "former things," then we can truly follow his way, and "be made new in the attitude of [our] minds; and to put on the new self" (Eph. 4:23, 24)—an inner self which, uncluttered and unmarred by the old data, is a beautiful reflection of our Maker.

HOW TO SIMPLIFY YOUR WARDROBE

In teaching seminars, I find that most women are collectors. They are collectors of old data—old habits, attitudes, and responses. And they are collectors of clothes. In fact, it seems to me the more insecure a woman is, the more clothes she tends to collect (as though this will help her to find herself).

In the earlier portion of this chapter, we talked about getting rid of "old tapes," and I've noticed that as a woman sheds old belief systems and feelings of unworthiness or low self-esteem, she is also liberated from such ideas as not being "good enough" to dress nicely, not being "worthy" of a new pair of shoes.

The opposite is also true: when a woman gives herself permission to look her very best, she feels better about herself. The language of clothes works on the wearer of the clothes, as well as the beholder! There's a looking glass or mirror effect as your attractive appearance brings a positive response from the beholder, which makes you feel and look still more attractive.

In previous chapters, we've told you how to use your body type, your personality style type, and your best colors to create your own unique visual image. But perhaps you're wondering just how to begin. Relax. I'm not going to tell you to throw everything away! Instead, let's start with what you have.

Do you, by any chance, have clothes in your own closet, clothes in another closet of the house (or the attic or garage), and clothes in the coat closet as well? Some of us keep clothes as a scrapbook of our lives, a collection of memorabilia. Think about this as you go over your clothes and ask yourself if you really need to retain that memory. (If you must, keep it apart from your working wardrobe.)

And if your own closet reveals clothes jammed together on the rod, overflowing the shelves, piled higher and deeper on the floor, don't despair. I've seen closets which made Fibber McGee's look like the epitome of organization. It *is* possible to bring order to your closet, no matter how hopeless it might seem to you.

Are you feeling a bit nervous about this project? Congratulations; you're normal! My clients all tell me they feel uneasy, apprehensive, and foolish about "mistake" purchases.

They also tell me when they're through, the sense of relief is enormous.

Select a time to work on your closet when you have several hours alone. (Possibly you'll want one good friend on hand.) Unplug the telephone or put it in the refrigerator so you won't be interrupted.

Just as we took an internal inventory, let's take everything out of the closet. Sort it into categories: blouses, skirts, dresses, pants, jackets.

And incidentally, while your closet is empty, why not seize this opportunity to paint the interior white? A fresh closet will do wonders for your morale, and enable you to see each garment and its color clearly. If it's dark inside, you might also install a battery-powered light.

Your battle plan now is to trim your wardrobe down to a point where you're in control of it, rather than having it control you. Remember, it's much easier to keep a two-bedroom house than a ten-bedroom mansion. (Besides, I find most women wear 20 percent of their wardrobe 80 percent of the time.)

With this in mind, your goal will not be to have a lot of *clothes*, but to have clothes which "intermix" well, to create a lot of different *outfits*.

Now, standing in front of a full-length mirror, slip into each individual garment. Be sure to try on your favorites. Notice how you feel in them, the pleasure of wearing something great. Resolve that this is the feeling you'll look for in everything you buy from now on. (I do want to caution you, however, from my own experience, that if you carry perfectionism to the extreme, it can be ridiculous; you'll never buy anything.)

It's a good idea to start with your suits or the most costly garments you might plan to build a wardrobe around.

As you look in the mirror, ask yourself seven questions:

1. Does it fit? (See chapter 2, plus "Fitting Details," below.)
2. Does the color truly flatter me? (Am I more radiant when I wear it?)
3. Is it my style type? (Is it really an expression of me?)
4. Is it the best image? (Am I projecting what I want others to see in me? Am I using wisely the language of clothes? Does a stiff fabric, for instance, project a lack of approachability?)
5. Are there occasions in my life for which this garment is appropriate?
6. Is it hopelessly outdated? Did I buy into a short-lived fashion which looks silly today?
7. And (*most* important): How do I feel when I put on this garment? Do I feel wonderful, or is it somehow wrong?

FITTING DETAILS

- One quarter inch of your blouse sleeve should show beneath the hem of your jacket sleeve.

- Look for shoulder seams which fit and don't hang off your shoulder.
- Your pants should cover the instep of your shoe or top of the heel if pants are narrow. (Pants too short? Tuck them into boots.)
- Your blouse sleeve should cover your wrist bone. (If not, fill in with jewelry.)
- Watch for a smooth fit across the back.
- Be sure the collar doesn't stand away from your neck.
- If you have a marked indentation below your collar bones, padding can be added to a jacket or dress.
- Be sure shoulder pads are properly placed.
- Be careful of puckering in the front of a garment when it's buttoned.
- If the hem isn't even, redo it.
- Seek a flattering hem length. (To slenderize legs, hem should never end at the widest part of your calf. The reverse is true if you wish thin legs to appear heavier.)
- A coat sleeve should touch the wrist bone when the arm is bent.
- Be sure a full-length coat is long enough to cover your skirt.
- Slacks should fit comfortably in the crotch—not hang below or be so tight that they pull.
- Waistband should hold skirt in place, but not so tightly that it pulls out of shape.
- When you try on a belted dress, be certain the waist hits your natural waist, not below or above.

If you can't answer a hearty yes to all questions except the sixth, that dress—or that blouse—should go.

Generally a good indication that something is wrong is that you haven't worn a garment for a year or more. Chances are this means something is wrong about the color, style, fit, or line, and you probably won't wear it in the next year—or two, or five, either.

On the other hand, if a garment is right in all those respects, try to determine what keeps you from wearing it. Is it too tight in certain areas? Does the label feel scratchy? Is it too revealing? Zero in on the problem and correct it.

It's hard for many of us to be ruthless about cleaning out our closets. (Having a trusted friend with you might give you courage— as well as an extra pair of unbiased eyes!) Every week I hear excuses, such as:

1. "My size keeps changing."

But if you haven't lost the desired amount of weight in three years of trying, I must be honest with you: chances are you're not going to. If you don't like the limit of three years, try for five. But don't be like the women I see who keep things from twenty years ago, thinking someday they'll squeeze back into them.

Instead, use the principles of body and line to "dress thinner" and look great today. Dress for now, not for that twenty-pound-lighter day that's over the rainbow somewhere. Remember, too, with your particular body type, you may already be at the weight that's right for you.

2. "If I throw everything out, I won't have anything left to wear."

Chances are, you won't throw everything out. And it's far better for you to work with a small wardrobe that makes you feel wonderful. It's possible on a limited budget of $200 to create the nucleus of a wardrobe if you shop carefully. I'll give you tips on this in the next chapter.

3. "I might need this if I ever paint the house—or for that special party."

If you someday decide to paint the house, one outfit is all you need. Put it in a bag on your closet shelf. Don't clutter your closet with your grubbies or your son's old jeans and T-shirts.

Put special occasion clothes and memorabilia which you can't bear to give away in a garment bag in the garage or in another closet. Keep its contents to a minimum, and away from your working wardrobe.

4. "I don't wear this because it doesn't go with anything, but it might coordinate with something I'll buy sometime—maybe."

If the garment is worth less than you'd spend to buy the extra items to make an outfit, it's not worth keeping. Be strong!

5. "This isn't anything special, but it's appropriate for church, a luncheon, a concert, or _____." (Fill in the blank.)

If it doesn't feel good, if it isn't becoming in color or style, it's a compromise. I see so many women who are lacking in self-confidence, and when they compromise on their clothing, they feed these negative feelings. Don't do it! Better to have one dress which makes you feel wonderful than twenty which are, "OK . . . I guess."

6. "I've only worn it once, and it cost me a bundle."

There is no such thing as a "mistake purchase." Someone will always be thrilled with it. A couple of years ago, I fell in love with a red silk fabric with green flowers. Every time I took a client into the silk shop, it caught my eye. Finally, I bought the yardage and had a dress made. I wore it once, and everyone told me how gorgeous the *dress* was. No one said *I* looked smashing. The red was too bright for me, and no matter how much blusher I wore, I looked washed out.

It sat in my closet until one day one of my consultants tried it on. She looked magnificent in it and bought it on the spot.

Someone else will love your "mistakes." And nowhere is it written that you must do penance for your errors by keeping them in your closet or, worse still, wearing them!

Are you ready now to look at your wardrobe objectively? Divide it into three groups: the "needs work" (repair, changes, alterations); the "if onlys" (if only this fit better; if only this wasn't such a bright pink, etc.); and the "love 'ems."

It's obvious what you need to do with the first group. As for the second, take a good look at the garments. What do they tell you about yourself? Clothes are often good indicators of feelings. Are there dreary colors which mirror depression or lack of self-esteem? Do too-bright colors indicate a need to relieve boredom? Does impulse buying reflect insecurities? Your clothes are your personal history and can teach you, if you'll allow them to.

Now it's time to get rid of the "if onlys." Perhaps you know that certain pieces will flatter certain friends. By all means, give them to them. Pack the rest up and ship it all to charity and take your tax deduction. (You'll give more away if you happen to be angry at the time. And that's not all bad!) Do it before you change your mind. I guarantee you'll not regret it.

One of my clients, who was recently divorced, found going through her closet a painful, tearful experience. There were twenty-five years of memories within those walls.

I encouraged her by telling her that cleaning out the old was the beginning of a new life, and indeed, it was. She's now happily remarried.

Another woman had dressd for her former fiancé, who liked a sporty image. But now she wanted to wear clothes which expressed the Romantic image that is really her. And as she cleaned out her closet, it became obvious to her that she got rid of a great deal more than just clothes.

Now that you've "cast off the old," here's how to go about reorganizing your wardrobe. I like to suggest approaching it as you'd plan a formal dinner.

Using the wardrobe analysis guide on page 141, list each of your major "love 'ems." Now, experiment with them. Try mix and match combinations, using different accessories. You may find you have many more outfits than you thought.

WARDROBE ANALYSIS

Item/Color	Style	Fabric	Coordinates with	Need to buy
Suits				
Blazers				
Blouses				
Sweaters				
Skirts				
Dresses				
Pants				
Accessories				
Shoes				

Also, make a note of which other items coordinate well with each garment. At the same time, write down what you need to purchase. From each item, snip a small piece of fabric out of a seam or hem. Place each sample on a safety pin. Use this when you shop, for matching and coordinating.

As you put your clothes back in the closet, try to arrange things so you can see them easily. You should be able to look, reach, and get dressed. If you must keep garments under plastic coverings, label them clearly from the outside. And be sure to label hat boxes and shoe boxes, as well. Or better yet, use see-through storage boxes and bags.

Slide out-of-season clothing to the back of the closet. (Or, preferably, put it in another closet.) Consider building an extra rod; it doubles your hanging space.)

Double knits can generally be hung normally, but knits which will stretch out should be folded in half, then folded again over a soft bar hanger. (You can pad it with fabric or tissue paper so it won't leave a mark on the knit.)

Do organize your clothes into categories: all jackets together, all pants and all skirts together, and all dresses together. Do this even with suits, so you'll be aware of the possibility of wearing the pieces as separates. When you hang your blouses, separate the dressy from the sporty. If you have a shelf near your skirts and pants, it's an ideal spot to store your folded sweaters. (Don't hide lovely things away in drawers where you forget them.)

The storing of shoes can be one of the bigger closet organizing problems. Ask my friend Susan. In her search for the perfect so-lution, she tried first an over-the-closet-door bag. It soon ripped from the weight of the shoes. Next, she bought an over-the-closet-door metal hanger. Every time she flung the door open, the shoes fell off. Then came the in-closet plastic bag with shelves. She had to unzip it each time she reached for a pair of shoes, and it quickly deteriorated. A stand (on which the heels of the shoes were sup-posed to hook) somehow regularly deposited all the shoes on the floor. Shoe boxes, though labeled, simply meant out of sight, out of mind. Plastic shoe boxes were too expensive. Her final considera-tion: a sturdy cardboard box with cubby holes. It sits high on a shelf. Try it. It works!

Hang all your belts on hooks or a special belt hanger, so they can easily be seen and not tangle; and line up your purses on a shelf.

And resolve today that you'll never hang anything which needs work (alteration, repair, or cleaning) back with your working ward-robe. A separate hook, perhaps on the back of your closet door, is an ideal place to keep such garments.

As you look at your closet and think about what you have, per-haps you're feeling discouraged over the mistakes you've made in your shopping, mourning that nothing you have is really right. Per-haps you're wondering how you can afford to have a wardrobe that's truly appropriate for you.

Let me assure you that you're not alone. I find that the women I work with eventually eliminate half to three fourths of their ward-robes. That's because all of us buy on impulse. We haven't enough sense of organization.

But take heart! If you really do a thorough job, you'll clean out three times more clothes than you need to replace. And the replac-ing can take as much time, or as little, as you wish. Some women want to do it immediately. Others take from two to five years. Set the pace which is comfortable for you.

And most important, as you work on your wardrobe, remember, in all his creation, God endowed us alone with the gift of selectivity. Use that gift well to give away all the clutter and confusion asso-ciated with your "old self" and to choose garments which echo the new peace and assurance and freedom of the "new creation" you are today!

BEAUTY IS DESIGN CHAPTER

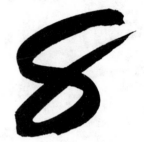

In our last chapter, we talked about eliminating the old data which has been cluttering our lives. But have you noticed that sometimes, when we get rid of something, no matter how painful it was, we feel a void which can be almost as difficult as the original hurt?

This was true for me after my divorce. I'd lived with physical danger and mental anguish, yet when it was gone, when I was by myself with my small daughter, I literally ached with loneliness.

I needed to think very carefully about a plan—a design for rebuilding my life.

I hope that, after reading chapter 7, you've allowed at least some of the old to "pass away." I hope you're freed of at least one old failure, disappointment, fear, hurt, or destructive behavior.

Now, how will you redesign or rebuild your life? With what will you fill the void?

Are you ready to assume responsibility for your behavior, calling on God to help and strengthen you, but avoiding the cop-out of simply shoving it all onto him ("God will do it *for* me!")? Can you also admit that you must begin with your attitudes toward yourself, which are inevitably reflected in your outlook and reaction to others?

Think a moment about what positive new qualities you would like in your life. What areas would you most like to work on? Then set a goal—or two, or three.

Here are a few suggestions. Perhaps they'll trigger other ideas for goals which are just right for you.

- Instead of drifting this way and that, have something solid to base my life upon.
- Learn to be more tolerant and patient with others.
- See each problem as a challenge for me to grow and develop.
- Love and accept myself.
- Make new and lasting friends.

Whatever your own personal goal, I hope you'll find it as encouraging as I do to know that, as you work toward it, there is a guide which has withstood the test of centuries. Often, we think of Scripture as a list of "shalt nots"; yet God never tells us what *not* to do without telling us what we *can* do. He knows that if we center on the negative, we're bound to fail. So he's given us specific principles to concentrate upon in replacing our negative behavior. And you'll find them all in the Bible. I find it truly is the book of life.

Suppose, for instance, that you are seeking that "something solid." Remember how the psalmist referred again and again to God as his rock? "He alone is my rock and salvation," he cries in Psalm 62:2.

In the New Testament, Jesus tells of the man who built his house on a rock, and when the rains came and the streams rose and the winds beat against the house, it did not fall. But the foolish man who built his house on the sand—well, you know the rest. (See Matthew 7:24.)

Later in the same chapter (Isaiah 41), God states, "For I am the Lord, your God, who takes hold of your right hand and says to you, Do not fear; I will help you. Do not be afraid."

Now, *there* is a promise to stand upon, to base your life upon!

But perhaps one of the other goals we suggested seems more appropriate for you. Whichever of these you seek, the key word is love.

In the great "love chapter," 1 Corinthians 13, we're told that nothing is as important as love—not prophecy or knowledge or sacrifice or—notice this—not even faith! And it concludes, "These three remain: faith, hope and love. But the greatest of these is love."

Moreover, this chapter states what love is not. It is not jealous, boastful, arrogant, rude, nor does it insist on its own way. Love is not irritable or resentful and does not rejoice in wrong.

Then it tells us what love *does*. It protects, trusts, hopes, perseveres, is patient and kind.

Not possible for you, you say? Well, that's probably true. But it *is* possible for God. You know, it's only because God first loved us that we are able to love him. And it's only because of God's love for us that we are able in any measure to love others. But if we truly focus on the freely given love of Christ and rest in it, then we can let that love overflow from us as living water. *That* is how you can love even the unlovable.

Of course, most of my clients are lovable, but now and then, there's a difficult one. And others ask how I can remain caring toward them. I have to point out that these people are reminders of the undeveloped areas which remain in me; therefore this "caring" is beyond my own ability; it is Christ's love flowing through me.

As you redesign your life, you will undoubtedly change your goals from time to time, and reevaluate them.

And do turn, again and again, to the Bible. It will help you to dwell on the good, the positive, and to grow in those areas which are honest and honorable, just and gracious.

One of my favorite biblical guidelines is Philippians 4:8: "Whatever things are true, whatever things are noble, whatever is right, whatever is pure, whatever is lovely, whatever is admirable—if anything is excellent or praiseworthy—think about such things."

And recently I found a simple but effective application of this passage. When I felt negative and tired one night as I approached a seminar, I asked myself, "If I didn't feel negative and tired, how would I feel? Why, I'd feel bright, alive, and shining."

And when I "thought about such things"—within a few minutes, I did indeed feel bright, alive, and shining.

You see, we do have a simple choice in our outlook as to whether we'll dwell on the negative or the positive. So the next time you feel "unlovely," ask yourself, "If I didn't feel unlovely, how would I feel?" The answer, of course, is that you'd feel lovely. Think about it. You have a choice!

You might want to thoughtfully read Matthew 5–7; 1 Corinthians 13; Romans 8:28; Acts 20:32; Psalm 119:114.

DESIGNING YOUR NEW WARDROBE

Just as your life needed filling in, redesigning after the old was eliminated, so, too, you'll see a void in your closet after you've eliminated what was not appropriate.

Here is a wonderful opportunity to make a design or a plan and to follow it . . . to truly be in control of your wardrobe, rather than allowing it to control you.

How, exactly, do you build a wardrobe which will really work for you, do the most for you, and give you the most for your money?

The first step is to take a careful look at your daily life. A good wardrobe is one which is flattering and appropriate on a day-to-day basis.

How—and where—do you spend your time? It's really a good idea to keep a log during a typical week.

Here's a chart to help you.

A WEEKLONG TIME STUDY

Activity	Hours Spent							
	Sun.	Mon.	Tue.	Wed.	Thu.	Fri.	Sat.	TOTAL
Out-of-home career								
Housework/cooking								
Child care								
Shopping								
Church/church activities								
Community activities/ organization meetings								
Theater/concerts								
Sports/recreation								
Parties								
Dining out								
Other (specify)								

Perhaps you'd like to arrange your activities in order now, beginning with those which occupy the most of your time.

1.
2.
3.
4.
5.
6.
7.
8.
9.
10.

Use this list in setting up your wardrobe budget. Probably the biggest and most important part of your life deserves the biggest portion of your clothes budget.

You may also want to consider your activities on a longer-term basis, comparing this year with last year. Think a moment about the times you felt you had "nothing to wear," when and where you felt underdressed or overdressed, uncomfortable or self-conscious.

Dressing does seem more complicated today than it was back in the days of the "basic" garment, such as "the little black dress." But I want to encourage you that, using the material from the preceding chapters, you now have greater freedom to find clothes which are appropriate and comfortable and much more becoming than those "uniforms."

We've worked out two basic wardrobe plans which should help you, whether your career is a very active one at home with your family, or whether you go out in the business world each day.

TWELVE EASY PIECES:
BASIC WARDROBE FOR THE WOMAN AT HOME

3 pairs of slacks
2 sweaters: cowl or turtleneck, cardigan
2 blouses: Revere collar, shawl collar
1 dress
1 matching skirt and blouse (patterned)
1 T-type top
1 blazer (to match one pair of pants)

To this, you might want to add two scarves and two belts.

If you limit yourself to two basic and compatible colors for the major pieces, let's see how you can mix and match.

Illustrated on the following pages are just a few of at least forty different outfits you can assemble from twelve basic pieces.

If you're careful about fabric and color, this could be a year-round wardrobe. Choose middle-weight materials. Transitional fabrics such as wool, jersey, challis, lightweight wool flannel, gabardine, rayon, silk, and crepe are wearable three quarters of the year. These colors are year-round choices: beige, black, camel, cocoa, medium and light gray, cream, navy, olive, periwinkle blue, purple, and red. And, of course, the style should not be too heavy looking or too covered up.

However, if you live in an area with extreme winters and summers, you'll probably need two wardrobes: one in winter-weight fabrics and one in summer weights (substituting an extra T-top for the cowl or turtleneck sweater).

Of course you will also need a winter coat, a raincoat, and three pairs of shoes: a classic pump, pants shoe or walking shoe, and sport shoe.

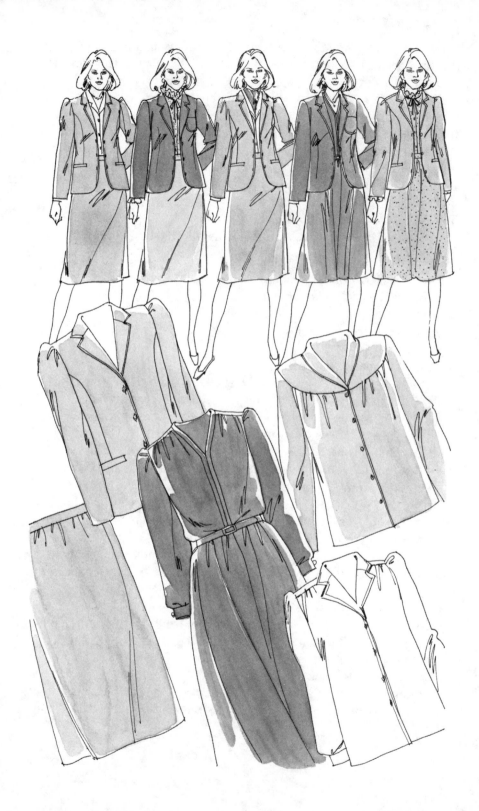

BASIC BUSINESS WARDROBE TEN TERRIFIC PIECES

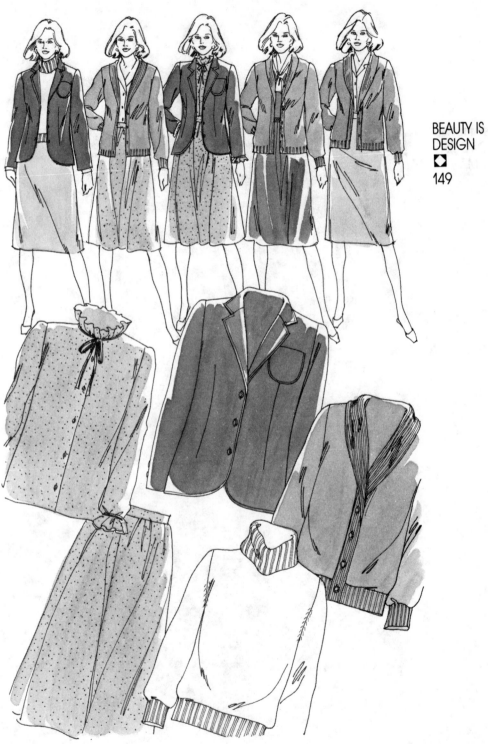

BEAUTY IS
DESIGN
◆
149

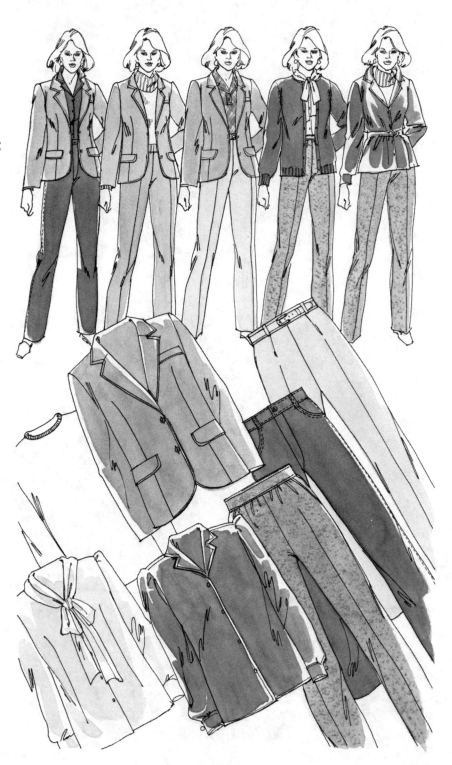

TWELVE EASY PIECES:
BASIC WARDROBE
FOR THE WOMAN
AT HOME

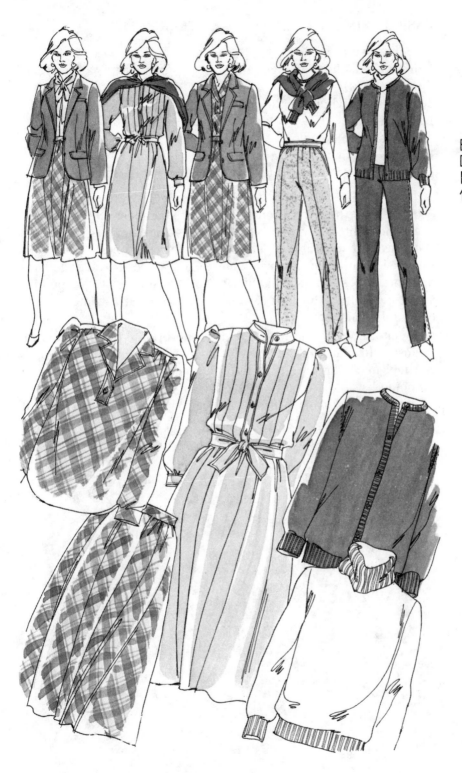

BASIC BUSINESS WARDROBE: TEN TERRIFIC PIECES

Two-piece suit
1 dress (capable of going from work to dinner with a change of accessories)
2 blouses: shawl collar, Revere collar
1 blazer
1 cardigan sweater
1 turtleneck (or cowl) sweater
1 matching patterned skirt and blouse

If you buy these components in, say, your best shades of red, navy, and white, they will mix and match into some thirty outfits. (I'd suggest two scarves and two belts for additional variety.) To this basic wardrobe, you will want to add a pair of walking shoes or pants shoes, boots (suitable for foul weather), classic pumps, and a neutral handbag. You will, of course, need a winter-weight coat and a raincoat.

Check the wardrobe which is most appropriate to your life style against your wardrobe inventory (chapter 7), making any changes you feel necessary. Use this information to make up a long-term shopping list.

Thinking on a shorter-term basis (and perhaps limited funds), if

JACKETS THAT MIX AND MATCH WELL

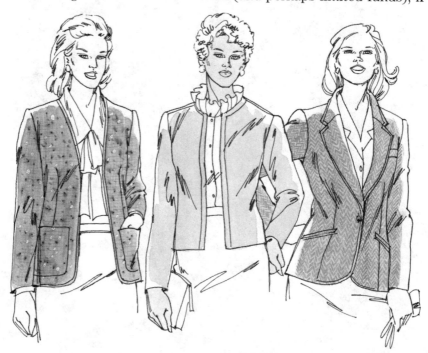

you can buy just one piece at the moment, make it a jacket and use it as a focal point for what you buy in the future. It needn't be the traditional blazer, but do look for basic styles with long-term versatility and wearability like the ones shown at the bottom of the preceding page.

Unlike the basics, the ones below don't mix and match well and you can't leave them open.

Another tip: To keep an up-to-date look, keep your eyes open for one current item to add to your wardrobe each season: a blouse or skirt with a "new" feel, but never an extreme look which will quickly become outdated.

Now what about color in your wardrobe? Since one key to mixing and matching is to start with two or three basic colors, which would be appropriate for you and your personal coloring?

Using these wardrobe plans, you'll have a multitude of mix-and-match possibilities. But you can give your outfits additional lifts at very little cost, or no cost at all.

Penny-Wise Perk-Ups for Your Wardrobe.
Try wearing a belt over a pullover sweater.
Blouse a cardigan sweater over a belt, leaving it unbuttoned at the top, for a sweater-jacket effect.
Add a sweater-vest to pants and a blouse for a pulled-together look

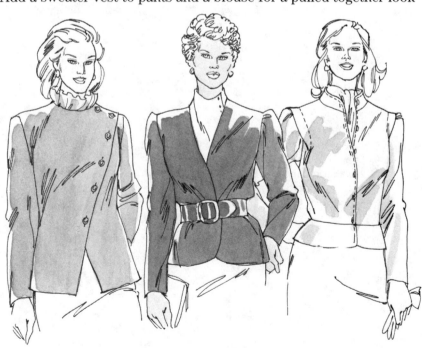

JACKETS THAT DON'T MIX AND MATCH WELL

SUGGESTED WARDROBE COLOR PLANS

	Basic wardrobe	Jewelry	Accessories	Furs
March: Bright Spring	navy, light cream, red	gold, diamond, pearls with golden hue, turquoise, coral, zircon	bone, camel, milk chocolate, navy	mink, ermine, squirrel, beaver, brown seal, stone marten with gold
April: Classic Spring	camel, light navy, peach	(see above)		
May: Gentle Spring	camel, light navy, peach	(see above)		
June: Bright Summer	light navy, blue-red, off-white	silver, platinum, ruby, emerald, turquoise, pearls	bone, taupe, gray, navy	mink: azurene, tournaline, autumn haze, palomino, natural; ermine; squirrel
July: Classic Summer	navy, dusty rose, burgundy	(see above)		
August: Gentle Summer		(see above)		
September: Bright Autumn	brick red, golden brown, gold	gold, emerald, light cream or ivory pearls, jade	camel, off-white, brown, beiges	brown Persian lamb, mink: ranch, autumn haze; leopard, sable, beaver
October: Classic Autumn	rust, cream, avocado	(see above)		
November: Gentle Autumn		(see above)		
December: Bright Winter	red, white, black	silver, platinum, pearls in white, gray, or pink tones, amethyst, garnet, sapphire	black, white, taupe, navy, gray	fox: white, silver, black; mink: black, diamond, silverblue, blue iris; Persian lamb
January: Classic Winter	blue-red, white, navy	(see above)		
February: Gentle Winter		(see above)		

which doesn't add too much warmth.

Experiment tying the bow of a blouse different ways: at the side, wrapped twice around the neck and knotted in front, or even tied at the back.

Use a shawl for dramatic impact.

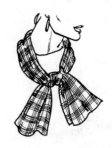

Instead of tucking a blouse in, wear it out, with a smart belt.

Try a hair-comb for a touch of color.

Hosiery in a color which coordinates with your outfit gives it extra zip.

Add a silk flower, for color and soft femininity.

Turn a collar up at the back of the neck.

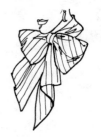

Turn up or push up sleeves for a sportier look.

Slip a long, contrasting scarf around your coat collar.

Give an old garment a new look with wonderful new buttons.

Make a "together" outfit of pieces in two different colors by adding a print which incorporates both colors.

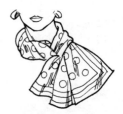

Cut extra hem material out of a skirt and have a self-belt made for a custom look or to replace the low-quality self-belts which come with many dresses and skirts.

Twist together two scarves of different colors; then tie them around your neck.

Turn your blouse collar over your jacket collar and lift them both up a little at the back of the neck.

Experiment with scarves. Here are just a few different effects you can achieve.

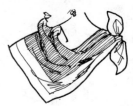

The Undercover Story. Now let's look for a moment at the undercover story.

LINGERIE

I must confess to you that my own underclothing is boring! During my years as a model, I learned that the least frilly and fussy are the best, because they don't leave lumps and bumps under your outer clothing.

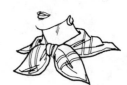

Do be sure, too, that your panties do not create lines which show under your skirts and slacks.

Your basic underclothing wardrobe should include:

- Panties, including some in "nude" color.
- Lightweight spandex brief (or control-top pantyhose) if needed.
- Two half slips (one light, one dark).
- Bras which fit well and support properly, preferably "skin" color.
- Full slip in neutral shade.

HOSIERY

With so many shades of hosiery on the market, sometimes it's difficult to choose. Ideally you will have:

- Several pairs of hose or pantyhose, one shade darker than your natural skin tone.
- Hosiery to match your special outfits (taupe, navy, black, etc.) Remember, your hose are an important accent to your outfits.

If your legs are heavy, they'll look thinner in darker tones. Lighter shades and thicker textures add weight.

DRESSING FOR "SUCCESS"

Although I do help many women (and men) dress for successful careers, this is a section of the book I want to approach very carefully, because I feel that true success is not of an outward nature.

There was a time in my own life when a motivation of anger spurred me on to seek success: I'd show "them" what I could do! Now I see success in terms of the great eternal hope which is mine. And, working from that core of peace and contentment, curiously, I am achieving more "success" in the world than ever before.

Actually, success in the world we live in can have many different definitions. What would it be for you?

Does success mean:

___Moving from the job market to a full-time career at home?
___Achieving a more active social life?
___Receiving more respect or love or attention or _____(fill in your own goal) at home?
___Becoming more effective in church or volunteer work?
___Reentering the job market after years of raising children?
___Teaching or influencing the younger people in your neighborhood, your children's school?
___Attracting a special man with whom you can develop a lasting relationship?
___Finding a new job or achieving a promotion?
Or _____ ?

Whatever you have checked or filled in, think about your goal; think about how you want to be perceived. Then go for it! Use what you've learned in the preceding chapters. Be sure to review chapter 1 and the language of clothes. Think about what you are saying to others, how you package yourself.

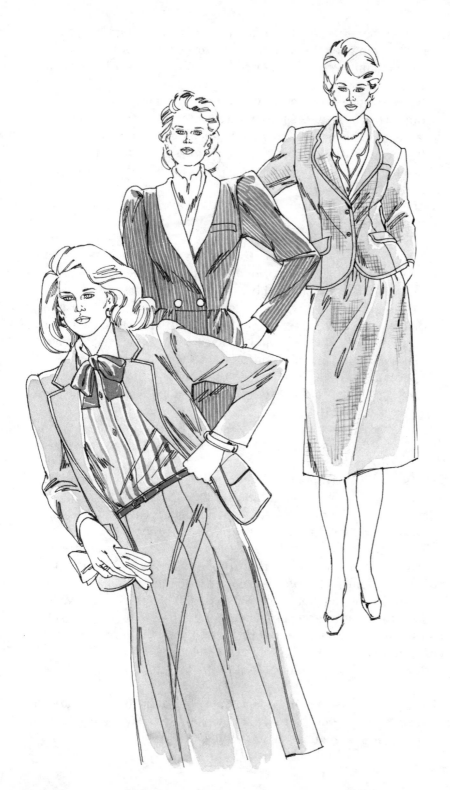

DRESSING FOR SUCCESS

Remember, too, to work effectively with body and line, to dress for the person you are, and to use your best colors. Dress to flatter your femininity and accessorize carefully. You will be believable, whatever your goal.

If you define success as advancement in business, remember that people who look successful and well educated receive preferential treatment. (This is true, as well, in social encounters.)

If you wish to be taken seriously, dress in a way that declares, "I'm important; I'm professional. Don't send me out to buy your ham sandwich."

The most common mistakes women make in the business world are:

1. Allowing fashion to decree what they wear—like the executive secretary who looks as though she's just jumped off the runway of a Bill Blass fashion show.
2. Dressing in ways which encourage men to view them as sex objects—with long, curly, bleached hair, low-cut, clingy blouses. (I've actually had management people request me to *do* something about employees who look like this.)
3. Looking too fragile and helpless—with ruffles and smocked-front dresses, cap sleeves, and a pale face which silently says, "Treat me gently!"
4. Dressing for their current position, rather than the one they want. (Chances are, the steno in polyester knit pants will stay a steno.)
5. As a reentry woman, failing to make the transition from being a cookie-baking room mother in a wrap skirt.
6. Overdoing the funky look—with dangling, clanging accessories, such as chandelier earrings; prairie skirt, boots.

How, then, do you attain the "look of success"? The main thing you are seeking is a professional, pulled-together image which will win respect for you, yet allow you to feel like *you.* Clothes can give you an edge; they can even make the first move for you when you feel timid, or are searching for exactly the right words to express yourself well.

Here are some specific ideas for "the look."

1. Always choose a matched or unmatched skirted suit. A pantsuit is not a good bet, even in a female-dominated company or even though male management says it's acceptable.

2. Choose from these preferred colors: navy, charcoal, medium gray, muted red, camel, rust, black, brown, beige, deep maroon, cream, dusty or heathery shades of teal, mauve, olive, taupe, green.
3. Avoid these colors: purple, green, mustard, very bright shades.
4. Keep your hair neat and smooth.
5. Wear a simple pump-style shoe; avoid clunky shoes.
6. Keep in mind that you represent your company or office to others. Impressions are lasting and part of your salary depends upon your being clean, attractive, professionally well groomed.
7. Avoid plunging necklines, clingy or tight clothes, sparkly fabrics, sheer fabrics, T-shirts, anything sloppy.
8. Keep your clothes in meticulous condition: shoes polished, spots removed, buttons firmly in place, hem secure.
9. Never allow a visible bra strap or panty or bra line.
10. Be sure your coat is long enough to cover your skirt.
11. Avoid bare legs, stockings with runs, reinforced-toe hose with open-toe sandals.
12. Boots are fine for snow or rain, but don't wear them in the office.
13. Avoid miniskirts.
14. Don't carry a canvas tote bag or woven straw bag.
15. Be careful of faddish clothes and extremes in pattern, cut, or design.
16. Try shirtwaist dresses or silk dresses with jackets, avoiding the too-fussy, choosing the understated.
17. The less you accessorize, the more credible you will appear. A woman who allows herself to become carried away with trendy scarves and jewelry reveals her insecurity. (Wear only one bangle bracelet [two will jangle] and no more than three rings total.)
18. Choose classic accessories which bring out the best in your clothes, make a positive statement about you, and are not distracting.
19. Almost every office has a "style"; be sensitive to what is considered a professional look in your company. Is it:

Super conservative: some banks, law firms, corporate offices. Wear matched suits, conservative blazers and dresses; dark and quiet colors. Avoid anything which detracts from the work at hand and focuses attention on you.

Middle of the road: most companies, corporations, schools, offices. Choose a more relaxed version of the conservative look, such as unmatched jackets and skirts, more casual jackets, sweater-jackets, a broader range of dresses.

Just slightly crazy: firms connected with show business and the arts; some fashion, cosmetics, advertising-P.R. companies. Almost anything goes here: the latest in funky accessories, ethnic looks, shiny and glittery fabrics; the wilder and trendier the better.

20. And be aware of special needs in certain businesses, such as:
    a. Dealing with the public: dress for the client.
    b. Sales: remember, you are your product. Adjust your clothes to one step above buyer's level. (For instance, if your client wears pants and blouse, you wear skirt and blouse.)
    c. Real estate: dress to match the property. (Show your neighborliness.)
    d. The glamor industry: peopled with chic and fashionable women who are impressed with fashion.

SUCCESS IN ACTION

My files are full of exciting "success" stories.

Norma listened to my discussion on packaging and said, "If what you say is true, then do a new me."

She'd wanted a supervisory position with her firm for a long time. In fact, for fifteen years she was interviewed every time there was an opening, but never promoted. When she repackaged herself to look the role of a supervisor—in smart suits rather than fussy print dresses or pants outfits—the company president, not recognizing her, stopped her in the hall and welcomed her to the firm. And yes, she got her promotion.

Martha, at age fifty-eight, had been laid off her job, and she might well have been depressed, since she was handicapped with a withered leg. But she knew exactly what she wanted to do: to become a speaker and encourager to the handicapped. We helped her repackage and she is truly effective today in her new mission in life.

Eileen, a divorcee in her thirties, came to me before an important party. Could I help her look wonderful—and possibly catch the eye of some nice guy?

I took an existing dress which had flattering lines but was a bit blah, added a silk rose in her best shade of red at the waist, along with a tie belt. We gave her hair more curl around the face and suggested softer, less exotic jewelry. Sure enough, she met someone special. It's beginning to look serious.

And when I urged a male client to dress up to the level of his important customers, he bought a good-looking navy suit, white shirt, and regimental striped tie. A few weeks later he called, delighted, to tell me he'd snagged the $25,000 account he'd been working on for four years.

Another woman, a data processor and part-time college employee, attended my courses and realized she was not the dramatic person she was trying to be, but really a Romantic/Sophisticate. She gave up her shark-tooth necklace, learned to dress for the person she really is, and finds she's treated much differently. She's respected and many people think she's the manager of the department because she looks the part. She repeatedly says to me, "Thank you! Thank you for what you've done!"

MAKING SENSE OF SHOPPING

When we showed you the basic wardrobe plans, did you think they looked wonderful on paper and you'd love to have a few pieces which mix and match so well, but that *finding* them all sounds impossible for you?

I hear you! I realize I'm a professional and I've learned to go to my favorite manufacturer's outlets where I can find the appropriate colors and lines and know the price will be right. So shopping is not burdensome for me; but it took many years of practice.

Most of my clients approach shopping with an anticipation similar to that of going for a root canal. They put it off and despair of following a plan such as we've suggested. Is there hope, then, for the "average" person? There definitely is.

Start by collecting a fashion notebook, gathering clippings of things you really love. This will assist you to become acquainted with your own taste. Then, keeping your best colors and lines in mind, make out a precise plan. Do it as though you were decorating your living room. Specify a color combination and an alternate combination. List each item. Then, hold out till you find it. Don't compromise.

Don't use the excuse, "I can't find it." You can, if you're willing to pay the price—and I don't mean the money, but the cost of time. You must expose yourself to a large volume of clothing. It will take you days of shopping, and you'll seldom find everything in the same store. But you *can* do it, and as you do, it will become easier.

Of course, if you sew well, or if you have someone who can sew for you, life can be much simpler. After you make your wardrobe plan, you pick becoming styles from the pattern books. Then you concentrate on shopping for fabrics in becoming colors and flattering textures.

If time is a great concern (and isn't it for us all?), you might consider mail-order shopping. The Career Guild, for instance, offers middle-range department-store type clothing which is color coordinated and perfect for the woman reentering the job market.

There are also excellent mail-order sources for the handicapped. *Clothing for Handicapped People* lists these. It is available c/o Naomi Reich, School of Home Economics, University of Arizona, Tucson, AZ 85721.

A few tips for shopping by mail:

- Compare prices with similar goods in retail stores, weighing the time saved against the cost.
- Use catalog firms' 800 area code numbers so your questions can be answered immediately.
- When catalogs carry name brands, try the brand of garments on in a store to determine your correct size.
- Save all correspondence and receipts, in case merchandise doesn't arrive or you need to return or exchange it.

Another time saver, if money is not a problem: many better stores employ shopping consultants who will work with you from your wardrobe plan. Remember, however, they are salespeople and one store may not have all that you need.

Now, let's consider some of the nitty-gritties of shopping.

First, cultivate an awareness of the ploys which stores and manufacturers use to get you to *buy*. Advertisements can be beguiling. Use them for information; don't allow them to create a desire for something you really don't need. Tantalizing window and in-store displays are another device. Try to put on mental blinders as you walk through the stores! Notice, too, that most stores are laid out in a way calculated to create confusion (no longer are there clearly demarked central aisles), and a loss of your sense of time.

And have you found that just when you learn where everything is in a particular store, they completely rearrange the departments, so you must search and search?

When you're ready to go shopping, what should you take with you? First, of course, your list of clothing needs and your color palette. Also, take the snips of fabric of existing clothing which you placed on a pin when you did your closet inventory. Check to see that there's a mirror in your purse, so you can see the sides and back of a garment if the store doesn't have a three-way mirror. And bring an apple to eat, to keep your blood sugar up. (It's easy to become so intent in your quest that you shop past your usual lunchtime.)

You need to dress for the occasion, too. Be sure you look well groomed and put together. As we've already seen, you'll get much better service. I suggest wearing a flared or slightly gathered skirt which you can slip on and off easily and under which you can try a pair of slacks, if there's no dressing room available. (This is frequently the case at popular sales and manufacturers' outlets.) A buttonless light-weight pullover top is also easy to slip other blouses or jackets over. And be sure to wear comfortable shoes.

Now, here are some pitfalls you should consider, things which can sidetrack you from making good and lasting choices:

1. Fine quality. Yes, it's a pitfall if it blinds you to other considerations, such as style, color, fit. Never buy just because it's such good material or made so well.
2. Low price. A bargain is not a bargain if you need all new accessories, or, of course, if it isn't becoming or enhancing to your life style.
3. A friend's advice. It's fine to let a friend help by bringing garments to you in the dressing room. But be wary of advice, unless that friend understands you and your needs really well.
4. Buying at the last minute for an occasion. Do understand your own life style and try to anticipate your needs. (Sometimes it pays to "buy ahead" when you see that wonderful, timeless dress, even though you don't need it this year.)
5. Shopping when you are tired or depressed. It's as risky as going to the supermarket when you're hungry.
6. Buying on impulse just to be buying something, without regard for your total plan. (Be honest: how many impulse purchases did you find when you cleaned out your closet?)
7. Buying when you're rushed. Don't try to squeeze a major purchase into the ten minutes remaining before an appointment or at store closing time.

I remember rolling a lot of "don'ts" into one day as I was returning from a business trip. I was exhausted, but just had to stop at a special discount store in the area, determined that I *would* find something. I saw a silk dress for $34, and was so excited about the price, I chose to make a color compromise. It wasn't right for me, and ultimately I gave it away.

Here's a far better way.

A Good Shopping Sense

1. Keep a notebook with a complete list of what you need in your purse. (You never know what you might find when you're in a store to buy towels!)
2. Plan a two- or three-color wardrobe, using your color palette. (See chapter 4 for suggestions.) But be flexible within your palette. If this isn't the season to find teal, switch to another becoming color. (It's like planning a menu: if there's no broccoli, try cauliflower!)
3. Begin with neutral colors (especially in skirts and slacks), so you can easily coordinate outfits.
4. Use your color palette as you're shopping.
5. Use your style and line charts.
6. Try to buy one outfit at a time.
7. Consider existing accessories.
8. Create different looks with the same basic pieces.
9. Remember, cleaning costs can add 100 percent or more to the cost of a garment.
10. Think about cost per wearing of the garment. (A dressy eighty-dollar dress which you wear only twice costs you forty dollars per wearing. A two hundred dollar suit may seem extravagant, but if you wear it even once a week for four years, it costs less than a dollar per wearing.)
11. Consider fashion magazines a guide only. Choose what looks best on *you*.
12. Strive for a versatile wardrobe. If necessary, you should be able to go from one activity to another with perhaps only a change of accessories.
13. Buy the best you can afford as your "basics." Better-made clothes usually hold their shape and last longer.
14. Combine quality and lesser-price garments for a total look on a budget.
15. Wear the garment around the store. Sit down in it. Walk in it. How does it feel? Does it move well?
16. Stick to classic, beautifully tailored lines. Simple, chic clothing works anywhere.
17. Buy blouses and sweaters with other apparel in mind. Consult your list to see what you need to go with what you have.

18. Do some looking in finer stores to educate your taste and understanding of quality, even if you choose to buy elsewhere.
19. Always wait six months before buying into a new "fashion," because some do not last and very quickly look dated.
20. Look for seasonless clothes: fabrics which span the seasons, such as lightweight wools, fine jerseys, gabardine, fine cottons; colors such as navy, beige, red, white.
21. Be careful about sizes. (I can wear sizes as small as six or as large as twelve, depending on the manufacturer.) If a garment looks as though it might fit, give it a try.
22. Look carefully for good workmanship:
    - Generous seam allowances and hems.
    - Stripes and plaids which match perfectly at the seams.
    - Seams which are smooth, unpuckered, sewn with matched thread.
    - Buttonholes which are neither too large nor too small for the buttons and which are even and smoothly finished.
    - Zippers which are set in properly, zip easily, and do not pucker.
    - Colors in various pieces of an outfit which match perfectly.
    - Collars which lie flat and have a shape of their own.
    - Pockets which are sewn in properly and don't show through or look bulky.
    - Underlinings which help a garment hold its shape (particularly true of pants, fully lined jackets).
    - Raw edges which are finished to prevent raveling.
23. Don't settle for an "almost" fit. Buy the garment, but have it altered to fit properly. (See Fitting Details, chapter 7.)
24. Learn the difference between a fad (an isolated style which fades quickly) and a trend (which affects many items and is wearable by many).
25. Look for items which you will wear at least three years.
26. Choose clothing which can be accessorized several different ways.
27. Ask yourself, "Does this enhance my life style?"
28. Always look at the fabric content, specified on the label of each garment. Synthetics can be easy-care, but not as luxurious or comfortable as natural fabrics. Naturals are, however, more time consuming and expensive to maintain. Blends may give you the best of both worlds.
    Polyester blended with cotton or wool is crease, wrinkle, and shrink resistant, as well as stronger.

Acrylic adds crease and shrink resistance, strength, faster drying, softness.

Rayon with cotton adds luster.

Acetate with cotton gives a smoother feel, more luxurious look.

Nylon adds strength, spot and shrink resistance, pleat retention, faster drying, minimal ironing.

29. Check a fabric's wrinkle resistance: squeeze it in the palm of your hand, then release it. The material should not remain wrinkled and should spring back into shape.

Caviar taste and hot dog purse? I personally never pay the regular retail price for any garment or accessory. Most cities have bargain shops, factory outlets, manufacturers' warehouses, and recycled clothing stores which specialize in name brands. Look in your local bookstore or ask your librarian for a directory of the bargain shops in your area, such as *Save on Shopping: S.O.S.*, Iris Ellis's guide to factory outlets.

(ALMOST) EVERYTHING YOU NEED TO KNOW ABOUT FIBERS

Natural

Fiber	Basic attributes	The Good News	The Bad News	Uses
COTTON (jersey, pique, oxford cloth)	Smooth, durable, versatile, absorbent	Washes well, feels comfortable, retains color	Wrinkles readily, may weaken from sunlight	Blouses, skirts, sportswear, dresses
LINEN (flax)	Nubby texture, fresh crispness	Cool in warm weather, dries quickly, lint-free	Prone to wrinkling, may feel scratchy, requires careful (hand) washing	Dresses, suits
SILK (chiffon, crepe, organza)	Elegant, rich, smooth, soft, drapes well	Light but strong, dyes easily, retains shape	Requires dry cleaning or extra care in hand washing, rots from perspiration	Dresses, blouses, scarves
WOOL Worsted (gabardine, sharkskin, worsted flannel)	Firm, smooth, longer fiber	Tailors easily, holds shape, wears better than woolen	Requires dry cleaning, prone to moth attack, may be allergenic	Suits, slacks
Woolen (flannel, tweed, jersey, shetland, merino, Cashmere, camel's hair; can be sheer, crepe)	Softer than worsted, shorter fiber	Warm, generally comfortable, sheds wrinkles, slow to show soil	Generally requires dry cleaning or hand washing, may be allergenic, may feel scratchy	Sweaters, suits, skirts, slacks, dresses

How do you know what you're getting in some of the discount stores which cut the labels out of the garments? There is a way to find out. The Federal Trade Commission has assigned identification numbers to manufacturers, and by law, these numbers must appear on all designers' garments.

Here are a few of the ID numbers you might want to know.

Abe Schrader: RN15579
Anne Fogarty: RN48648, RN30669
Act I: RN36486, RN36789, RN51331
Anne Klein: RN40803
Beene Bazaar: RN42960
Bill Blass: RN38344
Bobbie Brooks: RN47302
Bonnie Cashin: WPL10113
Charlotte Ford: RN43163, RN50003

Synthetic or Man-made

Fiber	Basic Attributes	The Good News	The Bad News	Uses
ACETATE (Arnel, Celanese, Triacetate)	Soft and silky, drapes well	Resists wrinkles, holds creases	May require dry cleaning, color may fade	Lingerie, sportswear, linings for coats, jackets
ACRYLIC (Acrilan, Creslan, Orlon)	Similar to wool but shinier in appearance, soft	Moth-resistant, safe in sunlight, dyes well, blends effectively with other fibers	May stretch and lose shape	Knitwear, sweaters, fake furs
NYLON (Antron, Qiana, Zeflon)	Silky but slippery; knits may stretch	Lightweight, strong, resists shrinking, fading, washes well, dries quickly	Whites may turn gray	Lingerie, stretch fabric, blouses, dresses, hosiery
POLYESTER (Dacron, Fortrel, Kodel, Trevira)	Lustrous, slippery	Blends well with other fibers, wrinkle resistant, machine washable and dryable	May retain stains if not tended to immediately	Suits, slacks, dresses
RAYON (Avisco, Avril, Coloray)	Slippery, shiny	Blends well with other fibers, strong, versatile	Requires low heat for ironing	Sportswear, lingerie, blouses, dresses

Calvin Klein: RN41327, RN42642
Donkenny: RN43594
Evan-Picone: RN35685, WPL08582
Fredericksport: WPL06168
Geoffrey Beene, Inc.: RN33293
Halston Originals, Inc.: RN46616
Harvé-Benard: RN40679
Howard B. Wolf: WPL12324
J.G. Hook: RN51898
Jantzen: RN37966, WPL06979
Jonathan Logan: RN34972, RN44290, RN43232, WPL09442
Leslie Fay: RN43857, RN42711, RN16890
Lilli Ann: RN14962, RN29563
Liz Claiborne: RN52002
Oleg Cassini: RN32203, WPL09352
Perry Ellis: RN57272
Ralph Lauren Originals: RN56158
Sasson: RN54516
Stanley Blacker: RN30219, RN41550, RN55639, WPL11388, WPL11390
St. Tropez: RN55862
St. Tropez Swimwear: RN53466
Villager: RN17470, RN31242

Your local library may carry the *RN & WPL Directory*, which lists additional codes.

What You Should Know about Designer Discount Stores
- You can save 20 to 70 percent off list price, so bring your list of major wardrobe needs.
- Early morning and dinnertime are the least crowded times to shop. Weekends and lunch hours, plus some evenings, are peak hours.
- Check garments carefully. But even if it's an "irregular," the flaw may not affect the appearance or performance of the garment, and savings can be great.
- Educate yourself on current styles and prices before you shop. Know when a bargain's a bargain.
- If the idea of undressing in a common dressing room with others bothers you, wear a leotard under your clothes.
- If you like a garment but don't need it immediately and it's convenient for you to come back, wait and see if it's marked down in a week or so.

- If prices are beyond your budget (even though they may be less than half the retail price for designer clothes) remember that you may find similar quality for less in a resale or second-hand store.
- Accessory prices may not be discounted as much as clothing at discount stores (sometimes only 15 to 20 percent). You may save more at retail clearance sales.

Here are some other sources of excellent buys which you might consider:

auctions
estate sales
flea markets
garage sales
funky functional clothing stores
government surplus stores
antique and vintage clothing stores
rummage sales
thrift stores
drycleaners (most sell garments left over a year)
resale stores

The latter category, the second-time-around store, can sometimes give you an opportunity to buy designer clothes worn only once or twice by wealthy customers.

Tips for shopping at resale stores
- Get to know the store personnel. Explain what you're looking for and ask them if they'll contact you when these items come in.
- Remember, these stores take in seasonal clothing. The best shopping times are September and October for fall and winter; November for the holidays; April, May, and June for spring and summer.
- If the label is cut out of a garment, you can be fairly certain it was purchased at a manufacturer's outlet or discount store. The price, then, should be lower than what you'd find in such stores.
- Check the garment carefully for flaws and spots. (If you find one, use this to your advantage in bargaining.)
- Consider alteration possibilities. (I once made a jumpsuit into a dress by opening the inner leg seams.)
- If you find something that's just your style and color, inquire about the person who brought it in and ask whether she will be bringing more in. If so, ask the store personnel to phone you.

Be sure, too, to watch carefully for retail stores' sales. (If you hold off buying for a week each season, you'll save 15 percent on the first reduction.) Read the ads in your local newspaper to learn about special promotions and clearances. Get to know the lines carried by smaller shops which do not make "special purchases" but hold outstanding summer and winter clearances of regular merchandise. Ask when these sales are usually held and put your name on their mailing lists.

Now that you have some guidelines for building your wardrobe, I think you see that it will not be an overnight miracle. But I encourage you to believe that it can be done!

Ask the God of patience to guide you. And let this become a learning opportunity not to become covetous, to gain a new perspective, and to be a good steward of your budget as you work toward reflecting outwardly the beauty that is within you.

FINDING A BALANCE

CHAPTER

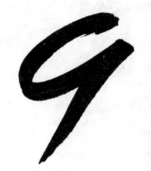

Where Are You Today?

There are so many exciting and effective ways to improve our appearance, it's easy to become totally absorbed in color and line and all the other tools which can bring about such dramatic change.

But it's also possible to concentrate so completely on our spiritual lives that we neglect our outer selves to the point that we come across to others as dull and drab.

What I urge you to seek is neither extreme, but a *balance*.

An Inward Look. Some of you, I suspect, have skimmed the "inner beauty" sections of this book and focused on the outer. To you, I would like to suggest that the total package is not complete—or, indeed, in balance—until you are willing to look at the innermost you.

Here is how Abigail Van Buren put it in her "Dear Abby" newspaper column:

"It's the glow from within that creates beauty. People are like stained glass windows; they sparkle like crystal in the sun. But when darkness falls, they continue to shine only if there's light from within."

I submit that this light stems from knowing personally the forgiving love of God. This is the radiance which no color or style can produce. This is the beauty which does not fade, but actually renews. (It prompts a son to tell a fifty-five-year-old mother, new in her knowledge of the Lord, "Mom, you're much better looking than you were ten years ago!")

Moreover, no matter how pretty we look, our *life* will never be beautiful if our innermost being is not transformed through a new birth. Then we are inwardly recreated and filled with the spirit and power of Christ because he is our very own Savior. Then we will look to God as our true source and meaning of beauty.

If this is a new idea to you, won't you, in the quiet of your own heart, ask a loving God to reveal his own presence in your life?

Consider these facts, as expressed in *You Are Really Somebody! ReAct*, published by Family Concern:

1. *God created me (Genesis 1:27). His creation gives me worth.*
2. *God loves me (Jeremiah 31:3). His love gives me belonging.*
3. *God planned for me (Psalm 139:16). His plan gives me significance.*
4. *God gifted me (Ephesians 4:7). His gifts give me competence.*
5. *Christ died for me (2 Corinthians 5:16–18). His sacrifice makes me completely acceptable to God.*

These facts establish my permanent worth. What God has accomplished cannot be changed. For me to refuse to accept, to ignore, depreciate, or deny these facts is a reflection upon God, a refined form of blasphemy!

In God's strength, I can now begin to be what I really am.

Indeed, you can truly be *Uniquely You.*

We'd love to talk more personally to you about this. If you have questions, or would like to learn more, write us at 24602 Raymond Way, Suite Q, El Toro, CA 92630, and we'll contact you.

If you are already a Christian, you know that the closer people look, the more beautiful you become—if they begin to perceive Christ within you, as a living part of you. Then your external beauty becomes a frame for the true work of art.

And we will *continue* to grow more beautiful! For God is preparing us someday to be the bride of the King. And in this process, more and more we both possess and reflect the ultimate in beauty—the very nature of God.

An Outward Look. I've given you many tools to use to become more physically attractive. But I know from my experience in teaching and consulting that some of you may not feel sure you want to use them. This is usually because you either don't want to pay the price or you don't want to change.

PAYING THE PRICE

By price, I don't mean money. I mean the cost to you in effort, in time, in pain.

What am I saying? *Pain?* Yes, in the sense that there is inevitably a certain amount of pain in growth. It's normal to feel you've made mistakes, and it's normal to feel pain as you walk through the steps of change.

This is certainly true of our faith, as James well understood when he wrote, "Blessed is the man who perseveres under trial, because when he has stood the test, he will receive the crown of life that God has promised to those who love him" (James 1:12).

And even Job in his profound misery could say of God, "When he has tried me, I shall come forth as gold" (Job 23:10, RSV).

It is also true that there must be pain in the sense of effort and trial for you to grow in your external beauty. So it's important to set goals that enable you to focus on the "gold" which lies ahead of you.

But before you define those goals, let's see where you are today. I suspect you've already come farther than you think.

Evaluating My B.Q. (Beauty Quotient) (Yes or No)

1. I'm beginning to understand that the way I dress and groom myself gives messages to other people about the person I am.
2. I've taken an "inventory" of my body: its basic shape and proportion. I'm learning some ways to make it look its best.
3. When I'm getting dressed, I think about how I want to be perceived.
4. I'm starting to see myself as the unique person God made me and learning to dress in a way compatible with the person I am.
5. I know some of the colors which are particularly flattering to me and in harmony with my natural coloring.
6. I'm working toward dressing in a way which reflects my satisfaction with being a woman.
7. I often receive compliments on the way I look.
8. I feel comfortable in my clothes.
9. I'm paying more attention to the impact which details (accessories, hair, makeup) make upon my total appearance.
10. I carry swatches of fabric and color with me to help with my shopping.
11. I truly want to make the most of what I have.
12. I've weeded out the unbecoming clothes from my closet.
13. I'm getting a feel for the "mirror effect": how looking better makes me feel better about myself, which in turn makes me look even better.
14. I have a closet full of clothes, but nothing to wear.
15. The various components of my image are beginning to be in harmony with each other. (I'm careful not to have beautifully styled hair but chipped nail polish, or to be well-dressed—except for shabby shoes.)
16. People sometimes think I'm a lot older (or younger) than I actually am.
17. I'm working to make my image compatible with my environment. (In a profes-

sional setting, my image is businesslike. In a home setting, my image is warm and relaxed.

18. If people who see me on a day-to-day basis bump into me at a party or in a restaurant, they often don't recognize me.
19. I spend hour getting dressed and still feel everyone else looks better than I do.
20. Salespersons in a busy store wait on others before they get around to me.
21. I've stopped impulse buying, as well as latching onto the very latest fashion as soon as it comes out.
22. People sometimes ask me if I'm feeling ill or unhappy, when I'm actually in great shape.
23. Strangers or people I know only slightly call me, "Honey," or "Dear."
24. I more often receive comments such as, "How wonderful you look!" than remarks about a specific aspect of my appearance. ("I love the color of your dress.")
25. I'm setting new goals to improve my appearance.

Score 2 points for every "yes" to questions 1–13, 15, 17, 21, 24, 25.
Score 2 points for every "no" to questions 14, 16, 18, 19, 20, 22, 23.
If you scored 42 or more, you have a top B.Q. Congratulations.
If you scored 32 to 40, you're getting there.
If you scored 24 to 30, keep working on it.
If you scored below 24—well, possibly you should reread the book!

Now, about those goals. Make them realistic and attainable. Make them consistent with your own personal values—not someone else's. But do make them. They're your motivation. Without them, you forget what you've learned. You simply drift along.

Here are some ideas to get you started.

GROWTH GOALS FOR MY APPEARANCE

This week	This month	Within six months	Within a year
Have my hair styled.	Shop at sales for a good suit and pumps.	Have longer, better groomed fingernails.	Firm up my hips and thighs by exercising regularly.

Now let's consider the other reason for not using what you've learned about looking better. It's not wanting to change. And curiously, I find that the more resistance there is to change, the more it's usually needed! The people who won't use their color palettes, the woman who won't discard the harsh, brassy-blonde wig—these are the very ones who could benefit the most from change.

WHY CHANGE? WHY TRY TO BE MORE BEAUTIFUL?
My own personal goal in life is to be of value to others.

And I sense that you, too, would like to contribute something worthwhile to other people.

One obvious contribution you can make is to add aesthetic significance to their lives. That's right; if you look wonderful, if your appearance is pleasing to the eye, then that in itself is of value to others.

But what if you have more than that to give to people? If you want, for instance, to teach them, assist them, minister to them? Well, how will you attract them in the first place if you don't look attractive? Like it or not, others find it hard to relate to a person who is very much off the norm.

Perhaps this book and the Uniquely You approach to working with your appearance has impressed you so much that you long to learn more and to share it with others. Are you also, perhaps, looking for the benefits of having your own business, the luxury of flexible hours, the opportunities to advance and reach your own goals, to achieve personal recognition? If so, I urge you to contact us regarding the possibility of becoming a consultant in the Uniquely You total image program. By all means, write us.

In working with believers, I am amazed at the insecurity they seem to feel about what they should wear and whether, indeed, it's all right to look their very best. When I've appeared on Christian talk radio, again and again women called to ask permission to look OK!

Yes! It's not just permissible; it's important! You show by the way you look that your life is in order, that you feel great about yourself, that you have that priceless commodity: hope.

Also, you will have more credibility if you look your very best, because it will be obvious that you could have been successful anywhere. Others will see that you didn't become a Christian simply because you are "weird," but because you believe there is a quality of life, a joy which only God has to offer.

The key, I want to emphasize, lies in balance. When we attain balance we will not become so obsessed with our outer beauty that we become vain and narcissistic. Rather, we will see it as a signpost, a means of pointing the way to God, our Creator, our true source and meaning of beauty.

ORDER YOUR OWN UNIQUELY YOU CUSTOM COLOR PALETTE

Uniquely You, the image consulting firm, would like to assist you on a one-to-one basis to compose your own personal color palette. This includes sixty to eighty-five fabric color swatches, a leatherette carrying case, a makeup guide, a personal wardrobe color plan, and a guide for coordinating your colors. To order yours, photocopy this page and answer the following questions carefully.

1. Turn to the color pages of chapter 4. Compare your skin, hair, and eyes to the color charts shown in the book. If there's any doubt or confusion, make a second choice.

   _____ color of hair, or possibly it's _____

   _____ color of eyes, or possibly they're _____

   _____ color of skin, or possibly it's _____

2. Drape yourself with colored fabrics. Do you and your friends and family feel you look best in:

   _____ off-white or cream   _____ burgundy or rust   _____ black or brown

   _____ dusty rose or peach   _____ soft gold or pink   _____ blue green or avocado

3. How do you see yourself?

SPRING	SUMMER	AUTUMN	WINTER
____ Mar (light/bright)	____ Jun (light/bright)	____ Sep (bright)	____ Dec (bright)
____ Apr (classic)	____ Jul (classic)	____ Oct (classic)	____ Jan (classic)
____ May (gentle)	____ Aug (gentle)	____ Nov (gentle)	____ Feb (gentle)

4. Your favorite colors? _____ _____ _____

5. Colors which bring you the most compliments? _____ _____ _____

6. If possible, enclose a color photograph (showing natural hair color, if possible). This may be a photo of you as a young person. We realize the color tones in the photo may not be totally accurate, but they will give a general idea of your coloring.

Uniquely You
24602 Raymond Way, Suite Q, El Toro, CA 92630

_____ Yes, please send my personal color profile.

_____ I enclose a check or money order for $35.00.

_____ Please bill my credit card: _____

( ) check   ( ) MasterCard   ( ) Visa   Acct# _____ Exp _____

Signature _____

_____ I'm interested in holding a **Uniquely You** seminar in my city:

   _____ color profile   _____ individual style, Line and Design Beauty Makeover

_____ I'd like to know more about inner beauty and its ultimate source.

Name _____   Address _____

_____ Phone: Day _____ Night _____
(city)   (state)   (zip)